Breakthroughs In Arthritis

Time tested and proven natural ways to successfully treat and prevent the hundreds of forms of arthritis and other related health problems.

William L. Fischer

Fischer Publishing Corporation
Canfield, Ohio 44406

Breakthroughs In Arthritis

ISBN 0-915421-15-1
Library of Congress Catalog Number: 92-073902

Printed in the United States of America

Contents

Foreword i

Introduction iii

Chapter 1
Understanding Osteoarthritis
and Rheumatism 1

Chapter 2
Diet, Nutrition and Arthritis 27

Chapter 3
Essential Fatty Acids and Arthritis 65

Chapter 4
Herbs and Arthritis: Natural Relief 79

Chapter 5
Arthritis and Exercise:
A Beneficial Combination 95

Chapter 6
Hidden Secrets to Overcoming Arthritis 117

Chapter 7
Gout and Bursitis 135

Chapter 8
Very Special Supplements 159

Epilogue 191

Appendix 1
Recipes to Help Overcome Arthritis 193

Appendix 2
Glossary of Terms 209

Appendix 3
Clay Resources 217

Appendix 4
Arthritis Foundation Chapters 218

Appendix 5
Bibliography of Selected References 231

Index 233

Disclaimer

This book is informational only and should not be considered as a substitute for consultation with a duly-licensed medical doctor. Any attempt to diagnose and treat an illness should come under the direction of a physician. The author is not himself a medical doctor and does not purport to offer medical advice, make diagnoses, prescribe remedies for specific medical conditions, or substitute for medical consultation.

Nothing noted in the text should be considered an attempt by William L. Fischer or the publisher to practice medicine, prescribe remedies or make diagnoses. Instead, knowledge received is strictly for purposes of education, and William L. Fischer takes no responsibility for its content.

Foreword

An elderly gentleman walked into his physician's office and complained of his left knee hurting. The doctor briefly examined the knee, made some notes on the man's file and then said, "Well, this sort of thing is expected. It's just a part of growing older."

The patient sat there for a moment, then replied, "Well doctor, my right knee is just as old and it doesn't hurt."

We consider arthritis as one of the complaints of old age. It is an unfortunate condition, everyone agrees, yet few among us consider it a condition we can escape. The truth is, though, that arthritis need not be an inevitable part of the aging process.

In many cases, we can prevent this painful joint disease and live our lives without being burdened by this often debilitating ailment.

Sound strange? I am sure that is not the way you have been taught to think of arthritis. In fact, with proper diet, proper exercise and a little determination, you may never have to know just how painful this condition — which seems to be reaching epidemic proportions in the United States — can be.

That may sound like a bold statement. Once you have read this book, *Breakthroughs In Arthritis*, you will understand just why I say this.

Breakthroughs In Arthritis gives those who suffer

with this disease hope. It gives those who have not yet shown any signs of the condition a chance to prevent it.

The most wonderful aspect of this book is its emphasis on natural means. Arthritis drugs are some of the most potent and dangerous a person can take. In many cases, they can cause a host of adverse side effects, some of which are as painful as the condition itself. The remedies provided in this book, however, explain how to rid your body of this joint disease without succumbing to such strong medication, without subjecting yourself to even more pain.

Breakthroughs In Arthritis is an encouraging book which will help every person who reads it, whether he has arthritis, knows someone who has it or is searching for ways to prevent the development of the condition.

I am delighted that a book of this sort has finally been written. It is long overdue.

Tom McCabe, RPH

Introduction

Your fingers ache, your back hurts. It takes a while to get moving in the morning because your bones don't work as well as they once did. This is what a mild case of arthritis feels like. Some people have arthritis so severe, however, that their fingers are disfigured and are practically useless. It is difficult for them to get up and move around — no matter the time of day — because the bones in their bodies hurt so bad and are so stiff. This is arthritis at its worst.

The term arthritis encompasses literally hundreds of different ailments, such as gout, bursitis, carpal tunnel syndrome and tendinitis. Explained in the simplest of terms, arthritis is a degenerative process of the joints which may be — but is not always — accompanied by inflammation.

The two most common forms of arthritis are osteoarthritis and rheumatoid arthritis. We will discuss these in more detail in the first chapter. These two conditions remain a mystery to the medical community; no one is quite sure what causes them.

And the diseases remain a mystery to those who suffer from them as well. For example, osteoarthritis can be merely a nuisance for some people for many years — but in others it can rapidly progress into a crippling condition.

Rheumatoid arthritis is equally puzzling. It follows an erratic course, remaining relatively minor for several years and then suddenly growing extremely worse, for no explainable reason.

These are only two forms of this common problem. Some of the ailments described in this book have little in common — others are closely related in cause and in the course of their development.

This book is designed not only to provide you with a better understanding of the major forms of arthritis; it was written with the intention of giving you control over your health and life once again.

This book brings you the best of natural medicine — herbal teas, massages, poultices — as well as other time-tested folk remedies to help you overcome arthritis.

We have searched the world over for the latest and most effective natural remedies. And we introduce to you several new breakthroughs in the forms of teas and other food supplements from such varied countries as Denmark, Japan and Germany.

It is exciting to start any journey — and you have begun the greatest journey of all — that of taking control of your health.

Good luck and good health!

William L. Fischer

Chapter 1

Understanding Osteoarthritis and Rheumatism

One national newsweekly magazine recently called arthritis "the nation's primary crippler." Indeed, the statistics are staggering. Thirty seven million Americans suffer with a form of this painful condition. This amounts to one in seven people. Moreover, one in three families -- one third of the nation's households -- are touched in some way by the condition. And the problem is not letting up. One million new cases are diagnosed every year.

Arthritis, additionally, costs the nation billions of dollars annually. Each year the country's businesses forfeit $27 million in lost work days. This, though, is only a fraction of the total $8.6 billion cost of arthritis, which includes the $4.4 billion spent annually on hospital and nursing home services.

A medical disease of such magnitude needs our understanding. What is it? What causes it? And perhaps the most important question of all: *Can we prevent it?*

This chapter deals with understanding the two most common types of arthritis: *osteoarthritis* and *rheumatoid arthritis*, more commonly referred to as rheumatism. Moreover, you will learn about several other forms of this condition affecting the body's joints.

Osteoarthritis

Osteoarthritis -- the most common form of this widespread medical problem -- is characterized by pain and stiffness in the joints. In most people, it is limited to only one or two parts of the body, for example, the fingers, knees, hips, lower back or neck.

The disease usually hits a person around the age of 50, but x-rays reveal that the deterioration may begin as early as 20 years of age in some individuals. About 90 percent of the population has some arthritic changes in their weight-bearing joints by the time they reach their 40s. After age 55, just about everyone is bothered to some degree by osteoarthritis, statistics reveal. Most people past the age of 70, in fact, have developed this ailment in their neck in varying degrees.

Women seem to be prone to develop it in their fingers, while men tend to get it in their hips. Osteoarthritis usually strikes both sides of the body. If you feel pain in your right knee, then you can soon expect the left knee to begin hurting as well. In general, the joint on the dominant side of the body is affected first.

A recent survey of people with osteoarthritis showed that 75 percent had the condition in their knees, 60 percent in the hands, 25 percent in the hips and a small percentage of people developed it in their ankles and shoulders.

Types of Osteoarthritis

There are two basic types of osteoarthritis -- primary and secondary. Primary is the variety that "just happens" for no apparent reason. You wake up one morning with a stiff, sore shoulder, but you don't know why. And the stiffness and pain stay with you. This is the type of arthritis people are referring to when they talk about the "wear and tear" on the body. It feels as if the joints are just wearing out. This common, simple explanation, though, does not answer the question of why some people acquire osteoarthritis and others do not.

By contrast, secondary osteoarthritis has a definite cause. It could develop because of a fracture, or infection to the joint, overuse of drugs injected into the joint, tissue damage caused by disease, such as diabetes, or by deposits of calcium in the cartilage.

Understanding Osteoarthritis

To understand osteoarthritis, you need to know how the joints work (see the illustration on page 12). Bones meet inside a joint capsule. The ends of the bones are lubricated and cushioned so they can slide past each other to assume their flexed or straightened positions.

The capsule itself is made of tough fibrous tissue. Muscles taper down to become *tendons* and attach to the bone at the joint. The ends of bones, located inside this joint capsule, are protected and lubricated by the *synovial membrane*. The end of the bone is covered by a smooth layer of cartilage which allows for ease of movement. Osteoarthritis causes this very important cartilage to flake and wear away.

In certain joints of the body, small pouches filled with a gummy fluid supply extra lubrication for the body's tissues. These are called *bursae*. When the bursae become inflamed, the condition is known as *bursitis*.

Looking at the structure in more detail we find that at the heart of the joint are two bones that meet and move. The tip of each bone is covered with a smooth layer of cartilage that creates a non-friction surface, allowing the bones to slide easily. The cartilage also absorbs shock.

The cartilage is affected in osteoarthritis. In the beginning stages of the condition, the swollen cartilage begins to flake. With time, deep vertical cracks appear. Cartilage cells attempt to repair this damage by accumulating around the cracks, but the cells are unsuccessful. Instead of helping the joint, this action puts it under considerable strain.

In an attempt to protect itself, the body then lays

down extra calcium at the outer ends of the bone where the tendons and ligaments are attached. Consequently, small bony spurs, called *osteophyte*, form inside the joints. They are most visible as the bony knobs at the end of the finger joints, called *Heberden's nodes*.

A jolt or twist may occasionally break the osteophyte off and then it moves about inside the joint space. Many people call this a *joint mouse*. It is possible for it to get caught between the two bones as they move, causing an extremely painful condition.

During this degenerative process, the synovial membrane covering the joint is affected as well. The membrane's blood vessels narrow, thus reducing the blood flow. As the joint is used, friction creates heat. The flow of blood is not adequate to dissipate the heat and carry it off. Moreover, when the joint is resting the membrane stiffens. This leads to "gelling" which makes the joint difficult to move.

Symptoms of Osteoarthritis

Osteoarthritis, a degenerative disease, appears gradually in the body, usually affecting only a few joints in its initial stages. Early symptoms include a dull pain and stiffness in one or several joints. This condition is usually worse in the morning and gradually eases as the day progresses. After a relatively short period of time, however, the person will begin to notice that the pain recurs throughout the day and then, for no discernable reason, disappears.

Moderate activity or stretching will ease the aches, but vigorous exercise increases the pain. For example, a secretary who complains of aches in her fingers will have difficulty typing and buttoning her coat as well as problems with other movements using her fingers.

As the disease progresses, the pain lasts for longer periods of time. Activities which once the person was able to perform easily, now involve much pain. In some instances, the person cannot do them at all. In addition, tenderness may exist and swelling may be present, as well as a redness and warmth around the joints affected.

In advanced cases of osteoarthritis, the joint may actually crunch when it is moved. This is called *crepitant*. The range of motion becomes limited and eventually certain joints may become deformed. Hands which are affected by this condition may take on a snake-like appearance due to the deviations of the small joints.

If the neck is affected by osteoarthritis, the disc spaces between the vertebrae are compressed due to a degenerative condition called *cervical spondylosis*. Indications of this process may be a pain which shoots from the back of the neck to the head or to the top of the shoulders. Pain may radiate to the hand. There may even be muscle weakness in the arm. This is caused by bony spurs which prompt compression of the nerve roots of the pineal canal.

In very rare cases, these spurs may compress

vessels carrying blood to the brain and prompt neurological problems and possibly even a stroke.

Obesity and Arthritis

Medical doctors have been aware of the increased incidence of osteoarthritis among the overweight for some time. But they could not say for sure if obesity caused arthritis. The extra weight on the joints, it was clear, aggravated the condition. For this reason whose who carry excess weight are encouraged to lose it.

Researchers now believe that obesity may, indeed, cause arthritis. Scientists at Boston University examined 1,420 participants of the Framingham (Massachusetts) Heart Study. They found that people who were overweight when the study began about thirty-six years ago were more likely to develop osteoarthritis than thin individuals involved in the same study.

In fact, the heaviest twenty percent of the women were twice as prone to this condition than the average participant in the overall study.

A similar study of more than 5,000 people, as part of the First National Health and Nutrition Examination Survey, drew the same connection between obesity and arthritis.

David T. Felson, M.D., who worked on both of the research projects, believes that the changes in metabolism due to obesity may influence the onset of osteoarthritis in some people. One of his reasons for this conclusion is the fact that obese people develop arthritis in their fingers, as well as their other joints, an area which would not be strained by extra weight. Research is continuing in this area.

Rheumatoid Arthritis

Rheumatoid arthritis differs greatly from osteoarthritis. Instead of affecting only one joint or the back, rheumatoid arthritis affects the entire body. For this reason, it is called a *systemic illness*.

Inflammation is a major factor in this type of arthritis. Not only do the joints become inflamed, but in many cases so do the eyes, lungs, heart, muscles and even the nerves. The inflammation begins in the synovial membrane which lines the joints. The membrane thickens and invades the cartilage, and eventually the bone. This process may damage the joints. Most commonly the wrists, elbows, shoulders, knees and the small joints of the hands and knees are affected.

A person with rheumatoid arthritis endures the pain of hot, swollen joints. But accompanying this is a series of flu-like symptoms -- chills, fever, loss of appetite, loss of weight, fatigue and a general malaise.

Although the symptoms usually appear gradually, the onset is sudden in about ten percent of the cases. In some people, it can develop as quickly as overnight. About forty percent of all rheumatoid arthritis sufferers are affected in the spine. It usually hurts when one moves his head. For some people, the pain is so severe that it even radiates to the forehead. Others cannot tilt their head backwards because of the pain and the accompanying tingling sensation in the arms.

In addition to the pain and malaise, many people develop disfiguring nodules under the skin. Ranging in size from a small pea to a pearly onion, these nodules signal the inflammation of a blood vessel. Most often they appear just below the elbow or over some other bony prominence. In some instance, the nodules may form over a bursa or tendon.

Rheumatoid arthritis is a potentially lethal disease, but fortunately, seldom develops to that serious state. About twenty percent of those who develop the disease recover from it with no adverse side effects. Another twenty percent suffer permanent joint damage. But the majority of those who get rheumatoid arthritis will be bothered by occasional flare-ups and periodic joint pain.

Unlike osteoarthritis, the rheumatoid version is a disease of the young, most often affecting those between the ages of 25 and 50. However, it can strike older people as well.

About seventy-five percent of those affected are women. Why women are more frequently the victims is a mystery. But medical experts suspect that hormones may play a part. Rheumatoid arthritis will frequently ease and in some instances disappear during pregnancy only to recur after the baby is born.

The Patterns of Rheumatoid Arthritis

Rheumatoid arthritis generally follows three basic patterns. These are *monocyclic, polycyclic and chronic.*

In the monocyclic, the arthritis lasts for several months at a time, then goes away. The polycyclic version consists of several shorter attacks of the rheumatoid arthritis. Between these attacks the person will feel fine.

Chronic rheumatoid arthritis, the most prevalent type, is one in which the person feels some type of discomfort most of the time.

In all three of these patterns, the disease becomes less aggressive as the years pass. You feel less tired and less stiff the longer you have the arthritis; the inflammation of the synovial membrane lessens and no new joints are involved.

Causes of Rheumatoid Arthritis

Doctors are not sure exactly what causes rheumatoid arthritis, although they do have several theories. Among these are two which have garnered the most attention:

1) A malfunction in the immune system which causes it to attack the body,
2) The aggravation of stress upon the body.

The first theory is the one most widely held by the medical community at the moment.

A properly functioning immune system produces cells which defend the body against matter that is foreign to the body -- such as viruses or germs. It does this through either innate immunity, in which the body instantly recognizes the foreign invader and kills it, or through *adaptive immunity*. This form occurs when the body is taught to recognize a virus through the process of vaccination.

But the cells can attack normal healthy parts of the body if they malfunction. These cells are filled with a digestive enzyme that surrounds and engulfs what your system perceives to be a foreign invader. When that happens you have an *auto-immune disease.*

The reason this set of events occurs in certain people is not clear yet. Researchers have found that in the chromosome of sixty-five percent of the people with rheumatoid arthritis, a defect in the area which controls the development of the immune system is present. It is practically never found in people who do not have arthritis.

Another possible cause of the immune malfunction is a virus which settles into a joint, causing inflammation. If it penetrates into tissue cells, the body's defenses may not be able to tell the difference between the virus and the person's own tissue.

Recent research is lending credence to the virus

theory. Researchers have identified a specific virus in some rheumatoid sufferers. However, before making any conclusions on the role of this virus, it needs to be confirmed in a larger group of people.

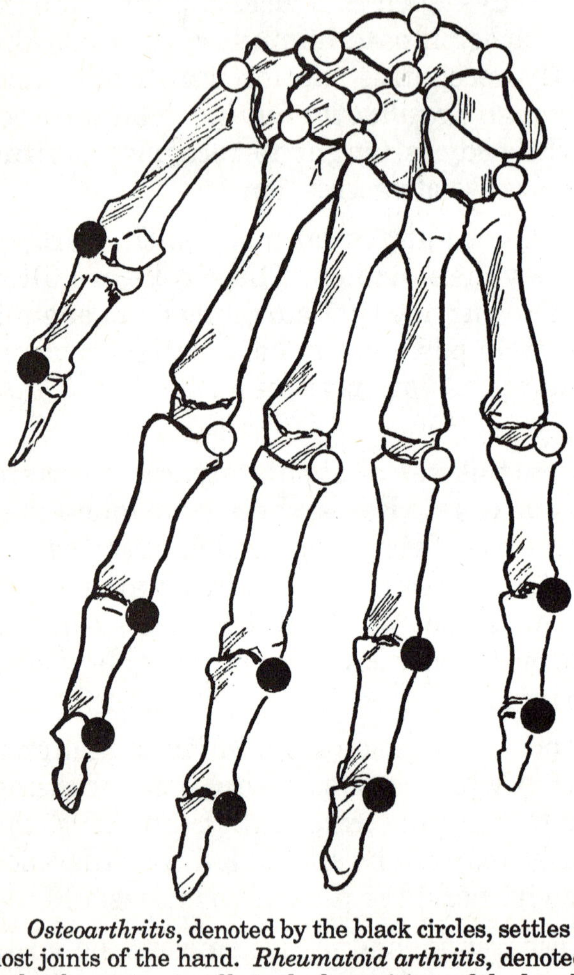

Osteoarthritis, denoted by the black circles, settles into the outermost joints of the hand. *Rheumatoid arthritis*, denoted by the white circles, by contrast, affects the lower joints of the hand and wrist.

Rheumatoid Arthritis: When To Seek Medical Attention

Rheumatoid arthritis, for many people, is a mild problem. But it can recur regularly and it may, indeed, escalate into a chronic condition. Below are four symptoms which may indicate your arthritis is worsening and may develop into a more serious condition. If you have any of these symptoms, consult your doctor.

* Pain, swelling, or tenderness in one or more joints.
* Recurrence of pain in the knees, neck, lower back, and other joints.
* Pain and stiffness when you get up in the morning.
* Recurring pain which involves more than one joint.

The Stress Theory

Doctors who research the causes of rheumatoid arthritis are learning that, in addition to an injury to a joint, infection, or a weakened physical state, the disease may also be caused by emotional disturbances.

Studies have been conducted recently to determine an association between the occurrence of stressful events in a person's life and attacks of rheumatoid arthritis. It appears that for about half of the people, a connection exists.

In one study, doctors discovered that stress precipitated an attack in almost fifty percent of the 293 people involved. In another project, doctors instructed rheumatoid arthritis sufferers to keep a "life chart." This is a record of their attacks as well as stressful events. In sixty-two percent of the cases, a relationship between the two was found.

Researchers are not sure of the reasons for the body's reaction to stress. However, limited work has determined that, for those who suffer with this disease, stress was a large part of their lives just prior to their first acquiring it.

Experts believe, also, that it is not the stress that actually causes the flare-up, but rather the person's reaction to and management of that stress.

If this is true, then you may be able to lessen the severity and perhaps even the frequency of the attacks by learning to handle the stresses of your life better. Doctors emphasize that a stressful event is not limited to unpleasant occurrences. Joyous moment, such as the marriage of a child or the beginning of that new job you always dreamed of, can be equally as difficult for the nerves.

If you suspect that your rheumatoid arthritis episodes are either caused or aggravated by stress, keep your own "life chart." It is easy to do. Get a calendar large enough to make notations on specific days. Keep track of your arthritis flare-ups as well as what happened on those days. There is no need to make a notation for every day, just those days when a bout of arthritis occurs. Following is a sample calendar. Page 16 can be removed for your use as a "life chart" calendar.

WEEKLY PLANNER	
MON	Finish Annual Report Staff meeting did not go well Pain in left shoulder and lower back
TUE	Dinner meeting with Jones & Company - new contract time. Back and shoulder pain worse this morning
WED	Got contract with Jones & Company Family night Did not notice pain when I woke up
THU	Company picnic No pain this morning
FRI	Raining very hard; must drive to meet new client. Shoulder pain very bad this morning.
SAT SUN	Cut lawn in p.m. - visit to in-laws in a.m. Going out to dinner with Joan and Paul; sitter hired. Pain in shoulder and back in morning, went away as day went on. None at bedtime.

WEEKLY PLANNER	
MON	
TUE	
WED	
THU	
FRI	
SAT SUN	

What To Do About Stress

If you find a correlation between your rheumatoid arthritis attacks and the stresses in your life, you need to find ways to either eliminate the particular stress or learn how to manage it more efficiently.

Not all stresses can be alleviated easily. Life consists of a series of stresses. While it may require discipline and determination on your part, the best approach is learning to manage your reactions to stress.

Stress reduction techniques abound in our tension-filled world. There are audio cassettes which can help you learn how to relax through meditation or other means. You might prefer reading a book on the subject; you can choose from a wide variety.

We will offer you just a few methods to introduce the ideas behind stress reduction. You may want to practice some of these. These ideas may also spark an interest and you may be motivated to seek other ways to handle stress.

Learning To Relax

One of the first steps in reducing stress is learning to relax. This can be achieved in various ways. One method teaches you to become aware of the parts of your body.

For example, just concentrate on your toes -- not on any of your problems of the day or on your pain. Tell yourself that your toes are relaxed. Believe that your toes are relaxed. Once you have felt the tension leave your toes, concentrate on your feet. Work up the body from there, to the ankles, calves, thighs, and so on, but do not leave that part of the body before it is relaxed.

This is not as easy as it sounds, but it does work for some people. It is a process that is accomplished only through practice. But once you have mastered it, you will discover that not only are you more relaxed, but you can better cope with the situations that arise.

A variety of this technique has been used successfully by many arthritis sufferers to reduce pain. For example, people with *Reynaud's Syndrome*, the condition which causes the skin color to change when exposed to cold, have been able to raise the body temperature in their hands. They concentrate and visualize they are holding something warm or that their hands are in warm water.

Perhaps your knee feels as if a hammer is pounding it due to the arthritic pain. Visualize that hammer, ceaselessly hitting your knee. Once you have that image firmly imbedded in your mind, visualize it slowing down. It is now hitting your knee less frequently and eventually it stops completely. For some people, this will lessen and even eliminate the pain.

Deep Breathing

Another relaxation technique is deep breathing. When a person becomes excited or agitated, he may involuntarily breathe deeply.

Controlled deep breathing can help you relax. Close your eyes, visualize something -- even a part of your body that is tense -- and slowly inhale through your nose until you cannot take in any more air. Hold this briefly. Now exhale slowly through your mouth. Repeat this three more times. Then breathe normally. This exercise should help relieve the tension in your body.

Routines Can Be Helpful

Cultivate a routine. This may help you cope better with the stresses of your day and, in turn, help to reduce the severity and frequency of your rheumatoid arthritis attacks.

While routines have a bad reputation as being boring and dull, they can be a valuable asset for an arthritis sufferer. Boring and dull can be a blessing. A routine gives a person the feeling of being in control of his life. If, for example, the first thing you do in the morning is make the bed, that is fine. That act establishes a sense of order in your life.

Be sure, in creating your routine, you give yourself at least thirty minutes each day to do nothing. Pick a time during the day that is the easiest to stick to. You may want to time it to coincide with your favorite television show; that way you have a reason to stop whatever it is you are doing.

This period of time should require little, if any,

physical or mental energy. It is the period of the day when you can just lay on the couch. Your body and your mind deserve this peaceful thirty minutes. And you will be surprised at your ambition, enthusiasm and energy once you include this into your schedule.

Other Related Diseases

Juvenile Rheumatoid Arthritis

About 250,000 children are affected by juvenile rheumatoid arthritis, according to the estimate of the Arthritis Foundation. The cause of this disease is unknown and, in fact, the three types now recognized may really be three different diseases.

About half of the children affected have the *polyarticular* variety. This means only a single joint is affected.

One third of those with juvenile arthritis suffer with the *pauciarticular* type, in which several joints are involved, usually the knees. This variety usually disappears on its own by the time the child has reached his teen years.

The remaining one-sixth of those affected have *Still's Disease*. With this type of rheumatoid arthritis, the child may suddenly become seriously ill, running a high temperature, accompanied by a rash and swelling of the lymph nodes. An accurate diagnosis may be difficult because the joints appear to be unaffected.

Systemic Lupus Erythematosus

Very little is known about the cause of this condition, and therefore, medical science has yet to develop a cure for *Systemic Lupus Erythematosus.*

In this disease, a process occurs where the body produces antibodies which may attack their own tissue. This process may strike not only the joints and the skin, but also blood vessels, the lining of the heart, lungs and other internal organs as well. Tissue destruction may also result.

Systemic Lupus Erythematosus is characterized by a unique, butterfly-shaped rash which affects the person's nose and cheeks. Joint pain is reported by more than ninety percent of those affected with this condition. Arthritis deformities, however, rarely occur.

Women develop this ailment more often than men. For every man who acquires this condition, eight or nine females do. While it is not considered a rare disease, Systemic Lupus Erythematosus affects about one in more than one thousand persons.

Doctors diagnose the presence of lupus by use of a blood test which reveals abnormal antibodies, a sign that the body is attacking itself.

Psoriatic Arthritis

Psoriatic arthritis was not recognized as a condition until the late 1920s. Very similar to rheumatoid arthritis, several joints become inflamed in this ailment, accompanied by pain, redness, swelling and warmth.

Most commonly, the smaller joints of the fingers and toes are affected. The nails and nail beds may be pitted with psoriasis. The fingers may swell greatly, causing the description of "sausage digit."

In the typical case of psoriatic arthritis, the person will develop psoriasis first. It takes another ten or twelve years for the joints to become painful. Those with the most severe skin problems are most likely to acquire this strange form of arthritis, according to one Mayo Clinic study. Once the disease is established, the skin and joint problems will then emerge and recede together.

Reiter's Syndrome

This is a peculiar combination of the following health problems: arthritis, conjunctivitis, or pink eye, urethritis (redness and discharge at the opening of the penis), balanitis (inflammation of the penis), keratoderma blennorrhagicum (a rash on the palms of the hands and soles of the feet accompanied by changes in the nails) and painless mouth ulcers. Doctors believe that the condition is transmitted through sexual intercourse and think it is the result of an infectious bacteria.

Ankylosing Spondylitis

The name probably is not familiar, but it is a condition that has been around since the third century B.C. *Ankylosing Spondylitis* is also known as *Marie Strumpell Disease*, named after the nineteenth century scientist who was the first person to fully describe the condition. The ailment is popularly called "poker spine."

In extreme instances of Ankylosing Spondylitis, bone forms between the vertebrae of the spine and eventually fuses the spine, skull, ribs and hips into a long bone, which cannot bc bcnt.

The condition seldom gets this severe, though. Most commonly, pain and stiffness occur in the lower back. The onset of the symptoms is quite gradual. As the condition slowly develops, the pain increases and the back may remain stiff for several days. Then, unexplainably, the symptoms disappear. This pattern will then repeat itself periodically.

The disease will eventually travel up the spine, and in about one-third of the cases, joints in the arms or legs become inflamed. Other symptoms include a loss of appetite and a corresponding weight loss, and an occasional slight fever.

As the condition progresses in a person, it may also affect the *sacroiliac*, the joint of the lower back where the small triangular bone (located just above the buttocks) meets the hip bone. Fusing may also develop in the joints where the ribs meet the backbone

-- both in the front of the body and in the back.

As these joints become inflamed, fibrous tissue grows from the synovial membrane and into the cartilage lining of the joint. The joint space will, over time, become filled with this material. At the same time, the bones near the joint also become inflamed and harden. Eventually, the joint space is transformed into solid bone. The vertebrae and discs of the spine also are fused together.

In its initial stages, Ankylosing Spondylitis is very painful. After the fusing has taken place, however, the pain disappears and only the stiffness remains. If the ribs and spine are fused, deep breathing is difficult because chest expansion is limited. In severe cases, the heart's aortic valve may not function properly and cavities may develop in the lungs.

In the vast majority of instances, the condition does not develop this far. Most people with the problem live active lives.

Most victims of Ankylosing Spondylitis are young men, some as young as fifteen years of age. It may remain undiagnosed, however, until the main reaches his late thirties or early forties. It is rare for this back condition to affect women and, when it does, the ailment never progresses past a very mild case.

Ankylosing Spondylitis appears to be a hereditary disease. In more than fifty percent of the cases, there is a family history of the disorder.

Arthritis Associated With Inflammatory Bowel Diseases

Arthritis can occur as a complication of some forms of bowel disease, most often ulcerative colitis and regional enteritis, a term which includes such conditions as *Chrohn's Disease, granulomatous colitis* and other forms of colitis.

Persons suffering with any of these conditions are more likely to acquire Ankylosing Spondylitis (see previous section for information on this disorder), or peripheral arthritis, an arthritic condition affecting the joints in the limbs or the spine.

Approximately fifteen percent of all ulcerative colitis sufferers develop peripheral arthritis, usually in the knees and ankles. Attacks last about four to eight weeks, but are infrequent. Similarly, Ankylosing Spondylitis is one hundred times more common in people with colitis than in the general public. The relationship between these two conditions is not clear.

Carpal Tunnel Syndrome

An inflammation of the tube through which the tendons pass is called *tenosynovitis*, and is usually the result of trauma. One of the most common types of tenosynovitis is *carpal tunnel syndrome.*

With this specific problem, which mostly affects middle-aged women, pain is felt with wrist movement, usually shooting down the fingers and up the forearm. The three middle fingers of the affected area, moreover, feel tingly and numb.

The size of the tunnel, or tube, which the nerve passes through is reduced due to the thickening of the tendon sheaths and arthritic changes of the wrist. The nerve, which is softer than the tendons, is subjected to considerable pressure and corresponding discomfort.

If pressure upon the nerve has been present for a considerable time, the person affected with carpal tunnel syndrome will notice a clumsiness when he attempts very fine movements. The person may drop dishes, for example. Pain is usually worse at night. The individual may be awakened by discomfort in the hand which only exercise will alleviate.

Chapter 2

Diet, Nutrition And Arthritis

Many nutritionists and medical doctors now recognize arthritis may result from unwholesome eating habits. Arthritis patients experience near miraculous results when they eat a diet void of processed foods and rich in natural ones.

Those afflicted with arthritis usually eat too many foods made from refined flour, too many sweets and too many of the wrong kinds of fats. For the most part, the typical arthritis patient's diet is rich in refined carbohydrates and lacking in the proper amounts of vitamins and minerals. The damage to the joints, due to this pattern of eating, does not appear overnight. It surfaces only after many years.

Damage has been reversed in people who eliminate or severely restrict their intake of simple carbohydrates and other processed foods.

The Start

Some physicians require patients who wish to alleviate their condition through diet to eat only uncooked, fresh foods for the initial two to three weeks. A person with severe arthritis is often recommended, moreover, to eat only these foods for up to eight weeks. Typical of the fare allowed during this period is fruits, vegetables, nuts and seeds.

Additionally, while on this fresh food diet, you should abstain from coffee, tea, alcohol, nicotine and sweets. Tea is particularly harmful for arthritis sufferers because of the relatively large amounts of tannic acid found in it.

The elimination of these foods helps to remove toxins, reduce synovial effusions and eliminate the fluid in the soft connective tissue of the joints. This diet strengthens the life processes of the tissues and increases the body's potassium reserve. Eventually, the centers of the nervous system recover, as do the endocrine glands.

Many experts believe that the typical rheumatic patient's blood flows sluggishly because of the clotting of the red cells stemming from low body energy. The raw food diet also helps to increase the person's energy.

After this three-week period, whole grains, cooked cereals (not of the refined quality), vegetable broth and potatoes boiled in their skins may be added. If, with these foods, you experience improvement in your condition, then you may add cooked vegetables, whole grain breads and unsalted butter (but only in small quantities.)

Once these foods have been re-introduced to your

system without any problems, you may then add mild white cheese, cottage cheese, yogurt and sour milk.

Arthritis patients are encouraged by the improvement in their health as they continue on this regimen and overcome the healing crisis of the first few weeks. Their confidence in the diet and themselves increases. A real enthusiasm for the dietary habits, as well as for life in general, is soon apparent. In some instance, this may be the first sign of any enthusiasm in these sufferers in a long time.

Permanent Diet

Several months on this diet proves, in the majority of cases, to relieve the arthritic pain and the other often crippling symptoms. For long-lasting freedom from this condition, though, the person must avoid processed foods and keep his diet rich in fresh, natural foods — raw fruits and vegetables and nuts. In fact, these foods should compose roughly one-half of his total intake of food. The other half should be made up of whole grains, cooked vegetables, lightly-cooked potatoes and dairy products.

Meat should be eaten only on rare occasions. Instead, substitute poultry or fish. The essential fatty acids of fish, in fact, are proving to be extremely valuable to the body's joints.

Fish contains an abundance of *EPA*, or *Eicosapentaenoic Acid* which, according to the latest research, is critical in alleviating arthritis. EPA is the only material that the body uses to manufacture prostaglandin which help to reduce inflammation.

If you feel that you would like to supplement your diet with Omega 3 oils, as they are called, there are now capsules available. Doctors are recommending these supplements to some of their heart patients as they also seem to provide protection from heart disease.

There are many Omega 3 capsules on the market today but the best that we have found is manufactured under the name *Salmon Oil.* It is available at your local health food store. Many mail order vitamin companies carry it also.

It would be wise, additionally, to add small amounts of *unrefined, cold-pressed, flaxseed (linseed) oil* to your diet. The best method of incorporating this oil, rich in not only EPA, but also other essential fatty acids, is to add a small amount, usually a tablespoon, to your cottage cheese, ricotta cheese or tofu daily.

Frank J. began using unrefined, cold-pressed flaxseed (linseed) oil to his diet. He had suffered from arthritis for over fifteen years. Within several months, Frank noticed a distinct improvement in his condition, something he had never experienced before. He not only could move his arms without as much pain, but the range of mobility of his limbs had increased dramatically.

If you are considering adding flaxseed (linseed) oil to your diet, be careful to use only that which is *unrefined and cold-pressed.* This method of processing ensures the essential fatty acids and other nutrients are not destroyed, as is done when oils are heated to extreme temperatures. If the flaxseed oil you buy does not say it is unrefined and cold-pressed, then you are not benefitting from it. This product may be found in your local health food stores or through a vitamin company's mail order catalog.

Recipes to help you enjoy variety on this natural foods diet are included in the appendix of this book. The ideas in this plan may be new to you and may take a while to get adjusted to; however, the rewards of the program are remarkable. You may enjoy freedom from pain, increased mobility of your joints as well as unlimited energy.

Fruits and Vegetables Fight Arthritis

Consider the fact that animals, which later turn up on your dinner table as steaks, pork chops or roasts, get their cell-building power from vegetables, grains and other plants. When you eat meat for protein, as most people do, you are really getting a second- hand source for cell-building. Balance your diet by eating plenty of good, fresh fruits and vegetables.

Most ailments, including arthritis, respond to the curative powers in fresh fruits and vegetables. Vegetables give us vitamins, salts, trace elements, chlorophyll and yeast without fouling our bodies with wastes and toxins. They also give us fiber. The walls of the cells of vegetables are made of fiber, which is indispensable to our digestive system.

Fiber works in the intestines like a cleaning machine, sweeping their walls. Vegetables are among the champions of nutrition. Putting meat, sugar, salt, fats and white flour on one side of the scale and fresh fruits, raw vegetables, honey, whole grains on the other, the balance is clear. The first group are full of wastes and toxins and poor in vitamins, enzymes, trace elements, mineral salts, chlorophyll and fiber — the riches you receive when you choose from the second group.

To protect the body's organs from excessive fatigue, aging and illness, it is wise to choose raw vegetables as often as possible. However, proceed with caution. Even the most beneficial foods, when eaten in excess, are harmful. Eat intelligently and and choose your foods carefully. Do not settle for second best but only the freshest vegetables and fruits. Do not soak them in water all day long; they will lose many of their minerals. Wash them just before eating.

Some of the fruits and vegetables that are especially effective in aiding those with arthritis are lemons, raspberries, grapes, currants, apples, pears, tomatoes, leeks, green beans, onions and celery. In addition, many folk remedies suggest that uric acid, found in gout, is lessened by eating onions and grapes.

A popular method of consuming fruits and vegetables these days is in juices, carefully made in a home blender or juicer, using fresh produce. Fruits and vegetables should be at room temperature before being made into juice drinks. The following drinks are believed to prevent the occurrence of arthritis and to aid in the treatment of the illness.

Anti-Arthritis Cocktail

Wash	1 tomato
	several stalks of parsley
	2 stalks of celery
Peel	1 onion

Put the above in a blender or juicer. Blend or juice to a liquid. Drink slowly.

Green-and-White Delight

Wash and clean	1 fresh artichoke heart
Wash and peel	2 asparagus stalks
	10 radishes
Peel	1 clove of garlic

Put the above in a blender or juicer. Blend or juice to a liquid. Drink slowly.

Berry/Almond Pick-Me-Up

Wash	15 Strawberries
	15 raspberries
Prepare	3 shelled almonds

Put the three ingredients in a blender or juicer. Blend or juice to a liquid. Drink slowly.

Hawaiian Surprise

Peel	4 slices of pineapple
Wash and pit	10 cherries
Prepare	3 shelled almonds

Put the above in a blender or juicer. Blend or juice to a liquid. Drink slowly.

The healing properties of vegetables and fruits won't work unless they are accompanied by a complete reform in poor eating habits. You won't overcome arthritis by drinking the drinks above unless you make a commitment to a more healthy diet at every meal, every day.

Preparing Fresh Vegetables

When preparing raw, fresh vegetables, which are extremely important in the first several weeks of your new diet, four basic rules should be followed:

1) Vegetables should be eaten as fresh as possible.

It is best to use organic vegetables whenever you can. Additionally, they should be prepared as soon as possible before eating, not only to avoid wilting and loss of juices, but also to retain a high vitamin content. Do not shred vegetables until you are ready to eat them. They lose their nutrients when they sit in the open air, shredded or chopped.

2) High quality is essential.

Leafy and root vegetables should be young and tender with little bruising. The higher the quality of the vegetables and fruits, the better the vitamin content. This, of course, translates into a better diet and more health benefits for you.

3) Clean vegetables thoroughly.

4) Choose well-balanced combinations.

Each meal of raw vegetables should, if at all possible, consist of a red, yellow and green vegetable. A therapeutic diet, such as this one, should also include plenty of green, leafy vegetables.

Arthritis Vanishes

An eight-year-old boy who followed this diet is no longer victimized by rheumatoid arthritis. "His arthritis had spread to every joint of his body," his mother explained, prior to placing her son on this style of eating. "Billy was in the hospital almost four months out of every year."

Billy's mom continued, describing the side effects that her son experienced from his various medications. "He developed stomach ulcers, internal bleeding and allergies."

But when he began eating differently, his symptoms not only eased but they eventually disappeared. "He has thrived," reports his mom. "no more ulcers, no more allergies but, best of all, no more visible arthritis. He is now able to gain weight for the first time since he was five years old. His weight never was more than thirty pounds. He now weighs fifty-four pounds."

The change in Billy was so remarkable that his teachers did not recognize him when he returned to school from summer vacation. And, best of all, he no longer takes any medication at all."

Billy's mother supplemented his diet with a special drink on occasion. This drink — with a multivitamin-mineral supplement crushed into it — provides the body with plenty of nutrients, something many arthritic patients are lacking. You may use this drink as a breakfast every so often, or you may want to top your whole grain, cooked cereals with it. The instructions are listed below.

Super Health Energy Drink

This "milkshake" is an excellent way for arthritic patients to supplement their diets with extra nutrients and energy. If you wish, you may crush a multivitamin and mineral table into this drink.

1 cup low-fat milk

1 tablespoon lecithin

1 raw egg

1/4 to 1 tablespoon brewer's yeast

fresh fruit, added to your taste

1 multi-vitamin tablet, crushed (optional)

Mix the above ingredients in a blender until smooth. You may want to use the smallest amount of brewer's yeast indicated and gradually adjust your system to the full tablespoon after several months.

When you are beginning your revised eating habits, you may want to drink a quarter of a cup of this super healthy energy drink throughout the day, to introduce your system slowly to the ingredients.

If you have problems digesting foods, you should consider taking only one tablespoon of this drink every forty-five minutes or so. To use as an addition to your morning cereal, put only one-quarter to one teaspoonful on your breakfast cereal at a time.

Food As Medicine

"Let food be your medicine."

A wise man, centuries ago, spoke this memorable phrase. The Old Testament contains references to this idea as well. Unfortunately, it was a thought which we discarded as society progressed. Instead, we turned to synthetic medications, thinking they were much better.

Research now is proving that this ancient statement is much wiser than we had ever thought possible. Foods, legendary for their healing properties, not only across the nation, but around the world, are once again being seen as a means of helping people retain and regain their health. Indeed, more than ever, it would be the wise person who lets food be his medicine. And this is especially so for the arthritic.

Chili Peppers

Take, for example, the chili pepper and cayenne.

Folklore always held that a drop or two of hot pepper extract would help everything from a sore tooth to conjunctivitis, as well as killing intestinal parasites. Chili peppers also possess a traditional reputation for curing arthritis.

Scientists no longer scoff at the use of chili pepper. The active ingredient in this food, and in cayenne, is *capsaicin*, which stimulates and then desensitizes the "warmth detectors" in the hypothalamus gland. Researchers have now found the neurological mechanism by which capsaicin suppresses pain. This substance induces a reduction in the nerve cells of a neurotransmitter called *Substance P*. Substance P relays pain sensations to the central nervous system. In effect, capsaicin "short circuits" the perception of pain.

Chili pepper essence is currently being tested as an analgesic (pain killer). A single injection of capsaicin eases certain kinds of chronic pain in guinea pigs for weeks, according to research conducted by Thomas Burks, Ph.D, and chairman of the Pharmacology Department of the University of Arizona Health Services Center in Tucson.

In fact, merely rubbing an ointment of capsaicin on the skin numbs pain. Dr. Burks is optimistic that capsaicin may be used as the basis of a drug to alleviate the pain of arthritis naturally.

How To Benefit From Chili Peppers

If you want to benefit from the natural medicinal

qualities of chili peppers, but are not a hot food fan, the following tips may help:

1) Eat a little bit of hot food at a time.

Scientists say just about everyone can slowly build a tolerance for hot, spicy foods — and even learn to love them. Just go slow!

2) Eat yogurt with hot foods.

Quenching the burning sensation with cool yogurt, a few sips of milk or ice cream, is recommended by many. The native American Indians always ate something cold with their chili peppers. This works because fat — such as from yogurt or ice cream — dissolves the capsaicin, according to the latest research. This helps to hasten the medicinal benefits.

Lowers Blood Sugar Levels

Another property of chili peppers is their ability to lower blood sugar levels. While this is good news for diabetics (some authorities suggest three capsules of capsaicin daily for diabetics), this is distinctly bad news for those who have hypoglycemia. Hypoglycemics are counseled to stay away from any foods with capsaicin, as well as the herbal capsicum formulas.

Some experts suggest those suffering from arthritis take two capsicum capsules three times daily with a glass of milk or apple juice. At the onset of this therapy, you may notice a slight increase in your pain, but this will soon diminish. It is important that you take these capsules on a regular basis to enjoy the lasting benefits.

Barley Shoots: Relief From Arthritis

The green juice from young barley shoots exerts a natural anti-inflammatory reaction upon joints, the latest research demonstrates. According to a presentation given at the recent annual meeting of the Japan Pharmaceutical Society, the powdered juice significantly reduced the symptoms of arthritis in laboratory mice.

Based on this and other significant findings, several manufacturers are now marketing products to bring you the lasting benefits of this plant. It may not only help relieve arthritis, it also may affect your overall sense of well being. Barley shoots have already aided many people in taking control of their health.

Richard K. discovered the powerful rejuvenating effects of this remarkable supplement. In 1974, Richard was suffering from arthritis which affected him so severely he weighed only 89 pounds.

"All the medication they gave me," he said, "only made my condition worse. I was in and out of thirteen different hospitals. Nothing, absolutely nothing, helped."

Then he discovered several reports on barley and

its ability to eliminate accumulated toxins from the body.

Today, Richard is sixty-two years old and literally has discovered a new life. He not only snow skis and skates, but this energetic man sky dives and hang glides. "I have never seen or used anything so dynamic," he enthusiastically says.

Most people begin with one level teaspoonful of the powdered barley shoots, mixed well with cold water or juice before breakfast. They also take another teaspoonful with water before lunch. They continue this daily routine for several days, and gradually increase the dosage to the level which provides them with optimum energy.

The key to barley's success is the balance it provides your body. This balance is indicated in its composition, provided below:

1) Live Enzymes

Enzymes are necessary for healthy cell life and in dissolving protein and fat deposits in the body.

2) Alkaline Composition

Many processed foods are acid rich. The shoots of the young barley plants contain an alkaline composition which balances this.

3) Chlorophyll

Associated mostly with the process of photosynthesis in plants, chlorophyll increases the body's tissue cell activity and normal growth.

4)Amino Acids

The shoots of the young barley plant contain eighteen amino acids that are vital for good health.

5)Vitamins and Minerals

These young plants contain a wealth of vitamins and minerals. The powder includes thirteen times more *Beta-Carotene* than found in carrots, sixty-five times the *Vitamin C* found in apples, and five times the *iron* of spinach. Moreover, its rich potassium content balances the sodium in our daily diet, which may help to lower blood pressure in some people.

Turmeric

You are probably familiar with *turmeric* as a spice; it is a member of the ginger family. But you probably do not know that this spice has shown anti-inflammatory capabilities.

In fact, results from the latest experiments show that turmeric achieves effects quite similar to the popular anti-inflammatory drugs, *hydrocortisone acetate* and *phenylbutazone*. Some authorities recommend one-half teaspoon of turmeric dissolved in fruit juice and taken twice a day — in the morning and evening — may help ease the inflammation of arthritis.

Moreover, you may be able to receive relief by using turmeric as a base for a paste to be applied to the affected part of the body and covered with a plastic sheet and then a towel. The directions for this paste are provided below. It may also be used to help ease the pain of contusions, sprains and fractures.

Turmeric Paste For Arthritis

2 teaspoons turmeric

1 tablespoon lime juice

Boiling water

Mix the turmeric and lime juice together with just enough boiling water to create a smooth paste. The consistency should be thin enough to spread easily on the skin, yet still resemble a paste.

Gently spread this paste over the inflamed joint. Then wrap it in a plastic sheet and cover this with a white towel to keep in the moisture and heat.

This may be kept on for up to one-half hour to an hour. If the burning sensation is too uncomfortable, remove it sooner.

Celery And Okra

Celery and okra contain valuable nutrients which have been known to help arthritics. An easy way to incorporate these natural foods into your diet is in the form of juice.

Celery is especially rich in Vitamins A and C, as well as the B-complex family. Moreover, celery contains large quantities of magnesium, manganese, iron, iodine, copper, potassium, calcium and phosphorus. It is also an abundant source of sodium which, according to some nutritionists, is exactly what the arthritic is lacking. But those with heart problems should use celery carefully because of the high sodium content.

If you plan to eat fresh celery, be sure that it is crisp. Do not eat this vegetable once it is wilted or brown. Do not store celery longer than three weeks in your refrigerator.

Juices For Arthritis

Some nutritionists recommend drinking two pints of celery juice daily as a natural aid to arthritis. Additionally, they suggest you supplement this juice with one glass of any of the following combinations made in the proportions indicated.

1)	Spinach	4 oz.
	Parsley	1 oz.
	Cucumber	3 oz.
2)	Grapefruit juice	8 oz.
3)	Carrot	5 oz.
	Spinach	3 oz.
4)	Carrot	5 oz.
	Beetroot	1/2 oz.
	Cucumber	1/2 oz.

Raw Potato Juice

Perhaps the idea of potato juice is new to you. There are many reasons, though, why you, as an arthritis sufferer, should be particularly interested in it.

The raw potato possesses sugars that are easy to digest. However, when the vegetable is cooked, these sugars turn to starch. Moreover, the potato contains an abundance of potassium, sulphur, phosphorus and chlorine.

Raw potato juice is an excellent way to cleanse the system of toxins and it has been an important part of folk medicine for centuries. If you have a juicer, you need only put the vegetable in it to make potato juice. Then drink it diluted to a half-and-half solution with cold water.

If you have no juicer, simply take a medium-sized potato, wash it and cut it into slices. Do not peel it. Place these slices in a large glass and fill it with cold water. Allow it to sit overnight. The next morning, before eating anything, drink the juice.

Some people find the taste of potato juice rather bland and enhance it by adding a little carrot juice. This is fine and may be added to suit your taste.

Tea Therapy

Many believe that the natural elements in herbs are gentle, beneficial aids to preventing and curing many illnesses, including arthritis. When combined with healthy, natural nutrition, herbs can heal and strengthen the body.

To prepare the tea below, use heat resistant pans or tea kettles, such as pyrex, porcelain, clay or stainless steel — never aluminum. Measure quantities carefully. Prepare the tea a day ahead, if you wish. After standing overnight, they will only be more powerful. Keep next to a window or any other cool spot.

With each use, take as much of the liquid as indicated, leaving the herbs in the liquid until it is gone. This tea therapy is recommended for three weeks, following by a one week rest period before repeating. The tea can be carried to work in a thermos. Herbs should be purchased in small to medium quantities and can be kept for a year. Keep herbs in cold, well sealed containers. To help measure, keep these ratios in mind:

1/4 cup = 4 tablespoons = 1-1/4 ounce.

Arthritis Tea (two day supply)

3 tablespoons each of Gorse flowers
Juniper berries
Huckleberry leaves
Horsetail (entire plant)

4 tablespoons each of Elder Tree flowers
Licorice root
Soapwort leaves
Nettle flowers

Preparation: Put 8 tablespoons of the mixture in a saucepan. Add 6 cups of water. Bring to a boil. Remove from heat, cover. Let steep until completely cool. Strain and drink three cups during the day. Follow the cure for three months. If needed, repeat 4 times a year at change of seasons.

Veal Broth

Consider veal broth as part of your dietary habits. According to specialists, it is a wonderful remedy for arthritis. In fact, those with ailing joints in their bodies need the joint material of the shoulder of young beef to help rebuild their own.

Veal broth is also an excellent natural aid to digestive disorders, problems with the stomach, and the glands.

You can make this delicious soup as a course in your regular meal or you can drink it as a nutritious between-meal snack. The recipe for this soup is given below.

Veal Broth

1 fresh shoulder of veal
3/4 cup apple peelings, 1/2 inch thick
1 cup potato peelings, 1/2 inch thick
1/2 stalk of celery, diced
1 small parsnip, diced
1/2 of an onion, diced
1 beet, grated
1/4 cup chopped parsley
1/4 cup okra, diced

Wash the veal joint in cold water and place it in a medium-size pot. Put in enough water to cover the meat. Add other ingredients. Allow to simmer for about five hours. Strain the broth and discard the vegetables and meat. You may drink the veal broth either hot or cold. Store in the refrigerator.

Nightshade Foods

Potatoes, tomatoes, eggplant, peppers and tobacco may seem like a group of plants with no apparent link. But they all belong to a family of foods called *nightshade*. This group contains substances which block enzymes in your muscles from properly metabolizing waste materials.

For many of us, eating nightshades posses no problems, but for many others, especially those who suffer from arthritis, as little as one service of these foods may precipitate a flare-up of pain.

According to Dr. Norman F. Childers, who discovered the connection between these foods and arthritis, the problem is one of toxicity — a type of slow poisoning.

These foods release toxins which initiate the stimulation of solanine, a crystalline alkaloid which festers in the joints and muscles. With time, this substance lowers the body's resistance and prompts the onset of arthritis, Dr. Childers says.

Only about five to ten percent of the general population possesses a sensitivity to the nightshade family. However, Dr. Childers' research indicates that more than seventy percent of arthritis sufferers found relief when abstaining from these foods.

One person helped through the elimination of the nightshade family was a gentleman who had been bothered for twenty years with arthritis. As he eliminated potatoes, tomatoes, eggplant, peppers and, as he stopped smoking, the painful daily realities of the disease disappeared.

The man explains: "For a time, I could not believe what was happening to me. It simply couldn't be that easy. But, in just three months, the pain and restricted movement from twenty years of arthritis were gone! And it happened *without a single aspirin!*"

The elimination of these foods (many of which are hidden in processed foods) is not a quick fix. The success of this plan requires a faithful aversion to potatoes, tomatoes, eggplant and peppers, as well as reading the labels of packaged food products. And, even with this type of dedication, it may take anywhere from three to six months before you notice improvement. But the results — less restricted movement and a lessening of pain — are surely worth the effort.

Arthritis And Meat Consumption

Many arthritis sufferers eat large quantities of meat. By contrast, a lower incidence of arthritis is found in vegetarians. This may be more than a coincidence.

Meat contains between twenty and fifty times more phosphorus than calcium. Phosphorus stimulates the parathyroid glands, responsible for the mobilization of calcium form the bones. This calcium is then available to be deposited around the joints.

A second possible source of excess phosphorus in the diet is carbonated soft drinks.

Eating less meat and eliminating or reducing your consumption of soft drinks while adding calcium and magnesium supplements to your personal health habits may be good advice for arthritis sufferers. Some physicians recommend between 800 and 1,000 mg of calcium and 400 and 800 mg of magnesium daily.

It is extremely important to take these two minerals together as they are bound together in the body. There are tablets available which contain both of these essential minerals in the proper combinations. They can be found at your local health food store or through the many mail order establishments available.

Nutritional Therapy For Arthritis

Some physicians and nutritionists are experiencing success with a nutritional approach to arthritis. Various supplements are being used, including *Vitamin E, Vitamin C, Vitamin P, Zinc, Pantothenic Acid, Bone Powder, Royal Jelly, Propolis, Apple Cider Vinegar and Honey.*

Vitamin E

Doctors are baffled by the ability of Vitamin E to relieve the pain of arthritis. Two Israeli physicians conducted a study in which they administered 600 I.U. (International Units) of Vitamin E to a group of arthritis sufferers. A second group received a placebo — a harmless pill with no beneficial qualities.

More than 50 percent of those receiving the Vitamin E, the doctors said, experienced a "marked relief of pain," while only one person on the placebo noticed an improvement.

Writing in the *Journal of the American Geriatrics Society*, I. Machtey, M.D., and L. Ovaknines, M.D., confess they do not know why Vitamin E works. They suggest, however, that the nutrient may act as an anti-inflammatory agent.

Vitamin C

Physicians also have recommended large quantities of *Vitamin C* for the relief of arthritis pain. The nutrient is essential in the maintenance of the strength and proper functioning of the body's tissues.

One doctor who uses Vitamin C treatments for his arthritic patients explains, "We take arthritics who are practically crippled and give them their health back. Even the worst cases are rehabilitated in six months."

He prescribes 10,000 mg oral Vitamin C daily, having his patients build to this amount slowly. At first they take one 500 mg tablet with each meal and before going to bed. They stay on this dosage for several days. The doctor then gradually increases the amount taken until his patients take five tablets (2,500 mg) four times daily. The physician also noted that as large as these doses were, very little of it was unneeded and showed in the urine.

Another study confirms the need for Vitamin C for arthritis sufferers. It showed that those afflicted with this disease required more Vitamin C before their bodies received enough to satisfy their apparent great need. If you take more Vitamin C than your body needs for normal functioning, the excess will be eliminated through the urine. This will not occur, though, until the tissues throughout our body are saturated with the nutrient.

A healthy person's tissues may reach this point with as little as 200 mg per day. In some people, though, especially arthritics, this point is not reached until 15,000 mg have been taken.

It is true that large amounts of aspirin tend to use up Vitamin C more rapidly. This may be why two researchers in Ireland discovered that Vitamin C deficiencies are not uncommon in arthritis patients. Researchers at Trinity College in Dublin, Ireland, have learned that those with rheumatoid arthritis may require larger amounts of Vitamin C in their diets than healthy folks.

They measured the amount of Vitamin C in a

group of healthy people and a group with rheumatoid arthritis. Of those with the arthritis, a full 85 percent had levels which were well below normal. In fact, the Vitamin C level was so low in these people that they qualified for a diagnosis of *sub-clinical scurvy.*

Vitamin C also enhances the effects of just about any medication — including aspirin. Researchers at the Simon Fraser University in Canada took human cells from the synovial fluid of healthy and arthritic people. They cultured these cells with a combination of aspirin and Vitamin C.

The effect of aspirin on the arthritic cells was good. It reduced the growth on an average of twenty-three percent. The addition of Vitamin C to the aspirin proved remarkable. *The cells did not grow at all.*

You may want to consider taking a Vitamin C supplement for your arthritis. There are several excellent brands currently on the market. We advise you to consider taking one which also contains *bioflavonoid.* This heightens the powers of the vitamin.

Vitamin P

In 1753, Scottish naval surgeon James Lind proved that scurvy, the leading cause of death of seamen on long voyages, could be prevented by providing fresh fruit to the sailors. At that time, Vitamin C was unnamed and unknown.

It wasn't until the late 1920's that Dr. Albert Szent-Gyorgyi, Hungarian physician and scientist, succeeded in isolating Vitamin C from oranges. Most authorities were satisfied that Vitamin C was the active element in citrus fruits. Dr. Szent-Gyorgyi continued his laboratory work and, in 1936, won the Nobel Prize when he discovered a group of additional elements in fresh lemons and green peppers. When these elements were given to patients, along with the Vitamin C they had been taking, the patients responded more favorably than when given Vitamin C alone.

These elements, called flavone glycosides or bioflavonoids, were named Vitamin P. The P refers to the strengthening effect these elements have on the permeability of the capillaries, the tiniest blood vessels. So far, researchers have identified rutin, hesperidin and citrin as bioflavonoids but there may be more.

Although many fresh fruits and vegetables are good sources of bioflavonoids, the elements are largely destroyed by cooking. It is in the white pulpy part of raw vegetables and the thin skin separating the sections in citrus fruits that you find Vitamin P.

In nature, Vitamin C and Vitamin P are found together; they work synergistically in the body. Each activates the other and together they are more powerful than either one alone.

The bioflavonoids increase the strength of the capillaries. Like Vitamin C, they are water-soluble and readily absorbed from the gastrointestinal tract into the blood stream. They exhibit no toxicity and any excess is excreted through urination and perspiration. Results of clinical tests on the preventive and therapeutic uses of bioflavonoids have been published in respected medical journals worldwide.

Because many infections and certain degenerative conditions, such as arthritis, are associated with weakened capillaries, the effects of Vitamin P become especially important.

Dr. James R. West, of the Morrell Memorial Hospital in Lakeland, Florida, treated a woman in her mid-fifties with bioflavonoids for her rheumatoid arthritis. The woman was afflicted in both hands, wrists, elbows, knees, ankles and her right shoulder. After two weeks, the pain had all but been eliminated and her blood pressure dropped to a healthy 136. After five weeks, her joints were moving more freely and she had a great deal more stamina.

Excellent sources of bioflavonoids include all the citrus fruits, grapes, plums, currants, apricots, cherries, blackberries, green peppers and buckwheat. Just remember that there is ten times the concentration of Vitamin P in the edible part of the fruit than there is in only its juice.

Rose hips are an extremely rich source of Vitamin P and contain thirty times more Vitamin C than oranges. Rose hips may be purchased powdered or in tablet form at health food stores.

Pantothenic Acid

Pantothenic acid, also known as Vitamin B5, is fast becoming a source of treatment for those with rheumatoid arthritis. This nutrient may be able to reduce the pain and stiffness of the disease.

Studies confirm that arthritics possess a lower level of pantothenic acid than healthy individuals. One study demonstrated that these people found relief from the painful symptoms when given injections of 50 mg of calcium pantothenate daily — that is 500 percent of the established U.S. Recommended Daily Allowance.

Another study, performed with oral supplements of the nutrient, produced equally impressive results. Those conducting this project learned that oral calcium pantothenate significantly reduced the duration of morning stiffness, the severity of the pain and, perhaps most significantly, the degree of disability to the arthritis sufferer.

Doses administered in this study began at levels of 500 mg daily and were gradually increased to 2,000 mg.

The current U.S. Recommended Daily Allowance for pantothenic acid is 10 mg. Dr. Roger Williams, who discovered this nutrient, considers this to be far too low. Despite this, experts estimate that most American receive only one-half to one-third of the current minimum guidelines.

Zinc For Arthritis

The trace mineral zinc is not one most people associate with arthritis, but it just might help with your swollen joints.

One study indicates that zinc may be valuable in treating the joint pain, swelling and stiffness of rheumatoid arthritis. Two groups were used in the project. The first was given zinc supplements, the other received a placebo. During the twelve-week period of the study, those receiving the zinc began to feel better. Their swelling diminished and they walked faster and their morning stiffness lessened more quickly than before.

Another study, conducted in Denmark, showed that those who took zinc tablets need less pain-killing medication than before supplementation. Their joints were not as swollen and were more flexible.

Bone Powder

A long-term effect of rheumatoid arthritis is *bone loss,* with the severity of it in some people actually resulting in broken bones. The drugs used to treat the condition — cortisone and other steroids — accelerate the process.

Until recently, there was little you could do about it. Now, however, researchers in England are optimistic that they may have found a way to prevent the bone loss — with daily supplements of *bone powder.* The doctors took seventy-two people and divided them into two groups. All of those in the study were fifty years or older and all were on steroid drugs for arthritis.

One group took six grams of bone powder daily, along with their medication. The second group took only the steroids. At the end of the year-long study, members of both groups were measured for height loss, a result of broken vertebrae. They were also measured for bone density.

The group taking only their medication lost more height and density than the group taking the supplemental bone powder. the bone powder provided substantial amounts of calcium and other minerals and trace elements.

And an added benefit was observed by those taking the bone powder. Their pain was not as severe. Those who did not take the supplements complained three times as much about back pain as those who received the powder.

Royal Jelly

Royal Jelly has been called "nature's richest health food" and it has been known to help ease the pain and discomfort of arthritis in some people.

You are probably not familiar with Royal Jelly. It is actually the food of honey bees and scientists now credit it with the creation of a queen bee in a hive. Bees — all of them — feed on Royal Jelly, a milk liquid, for the first four days after they are hatched.

However, after this, the supply is cut off to all but the queen bee. Researchers now have determined that it is this Royal Jelly diet which gives the queen bee her distinct size and superiority over the worker bees.

Royal Jelly contains all the amino acids essential not only for bees, but for human health, as well as ten vitamins and six minerals. It is this rich nutrient content—plus something extra which defies duplication — that makes it so wholesome for humans.

It may be its high pantothenic acid content which makes it the choice of many arthritics when in need of a pain reliever.

Janet M., 57, had been an arthritis sufferer for several years. In that time, her condition had gotten steadily worse. Of course, some days were better than others, but there were those days when it felt as if every bone in her entire body hurt.

One day she went into a local health food store to buy some vitamins. She casually mentioned her arthritis to the clerk. "Oh yes, I used to be bothered something terrible with joint pain," the clerk commented, "but not anymore." "Since I've been taking Royal Jelly, I hardly ever complain of arthritis aches and pains," she told Janet.

Curious, Janet bought a bottle of Royal Jelly capsules. She took them faithfully for several days. In that time, she noticed a slight improvement. It encouraged her to continue. Her husband scoffed at her, but Janet soon became convinced of Royal Jelly's effectiveness.

She found it easier to get out of bed in the morning. Her joints hurt less and she accomplished more during her day. Within several weeks, even her husband admitted there was a difference in her personality. She was more cheerful and more optimistic about life.

"I never would have thought that something that came from the beehive could be so beneficial to people," Janet said.

Royal Jelly capsules may be found at your local health food store. Be careful in choosing a brand, though. Do not select any which have been heated. This process destroys some of the nutrient quality and quantity.

Propolis

A related bee product is *Propolis*, the resinous substance gathered by the bees through the leaf buds and tree barks. It is the material the bees use to disinfect the hives.

Scientists believe, in fact, that *Propolis is the most effective natural antibiotic ever discovered.*

Propolis is rich in amino acids as well as the trace elements iron, copper, manganese and zinc. It also contains a wide variety of vitamins including pantothenic acid, or Vitamin B5, which has been shown to be an effective treatment for arthritis.

The medicinal properties of Propolis have been

known for centuries, especially in the treatment of wounds and of inflammation of all types. In Russia, during World War II, Propolis was used in treating wounds.

In addition to helping ease the symptoms of all types of arthritis and rheumatism, Propolis has been variety of conditions, such as inflammation of the throat and mouth, tonsillitis, and ear infections.

In fact, Propolis can be tried on any condition involving harmful bacteria, germs or viruses.

Propolis capsules can be found at your local health food store or through the many reputable mail order firms selling health products.

Apple Cider Vinegar And Honey

In the New England states, it is said that the use of *apple cider vinegar and honey* to help relieve the condition of arthritis is as old as — if not older than — the United States itself.

As we have already seen, honey products may be an excellent choice to supplement your therapy. They are naturally rich in many essential vitamins and minerals.

Similarly, honey contains the nutrients needed by your body. If you now use sugar to sweeten your beverages and in your cooking, try honey instead. The sugars in honey are products of a more natural form than those found in refined, white sugar. Your body will thank you.

Moreover, try using this New England folk remedy for arthritis. Mix two teaspoons of apple cider vinegar and two teaspoons of honey in a glass of water. Sip this slowly, as if you were drinking hot coffee. Drinking this mixture once a day may, indeed, lessen your joint pain.

If you like, you may add two teaspoonsful of honey to a glass of apple juice. Just be sure the juice contains no artificial sweeteners or preservatives. You can find this type of juice in your local health food store.

Arthritis
Natural Guide To Prevention and Treatment

Vitamins And Minerals	**How It Works**
Vitamin C	Vital to the maintenance of the body's connective tissue. Heavy aspirin use depletes the body's reserves. This nutrient enhances the effectiveness of any medication.
Vitamin E	May be able to reduce swelling and pain.
Pantothenic Acid	May act as an anti-inflammatory agent and reduce pain and stiffness of joints.

Calcium	Essential for proper bone growth and health.
Zinc	May help relieve pain, swelling of rheumatoid arthritis. May increase mobility of joints.

Other Natural Remedies	**How It Works**
Bone Powder Supplements	May reduce pain of rheumatoid arthritis and prevent bone density loss.
Propolis	A natural antibiotic, may reduce severity of pain.
Royal Jelly	May act as a natural pain reliever.
Diet	Stay away from processed foods and coffees, teas and carbonated beverages, as well as alcohol and wine. Many physicians cite a diet heavy in these foods with contributing to the cause of arthritis. Instead, eat a diet rich in natural foods, such as fruits, vegetables and nuts.

Nightshade Foods

Potatoes, tomatoes, eggplant, peppers and tobacco are all members of the nightshade family of plants that produce a toxic effect in some individuals, which may be the cause of arthritis. Stay away from these foods for several weeks to a month to determine if they are toxic to your body.

Chapter 3

Essential Fatty Acids And Arthritis

A friend of mine was traveling the highway when he noticed smoke pouring out of his car engine. He pulled the car over, opened the hood and stared. Not being knowledgeable about cars, he didn't know what was wrong.

After he had his car towed and checked out, the mechanic told him what was wrong. "All the oil leaked out," the technician said, "and your engine blew. It's ruined. You might as well buy a new car."

An engine -- any type of engine -- cannot run without oil. It needs lubrication to keep all the gears and its other complex parts running smoothly and efficiently.

The human body is very similar to an engine in this respect. The body needs oil -- and the proper types of oil -- to run smoothly. If it does not receive oil and the nutrients oil contains, eventually damage occurs.

While the body does not literally blow up, as a car may, it does, indeed, manifest the damage through one or more degenerative diseases, such as heart disease and arthritis. Unlike a car, we cannot run out and buy a new one once the damage has occurred.

What Kind Of Oil?

When we say the human body needs more oil, we do not mean that people should indiscriminately consume all types of oils and fats. Only certain kinds are required and are beneficial. Consuming the wrong type can be detrimental to your health.

We certainly do not mean to imply that large servings are necessary. Quite the opposite. When used sparingly, these oils provide your body with nutrients and essential fatty acids required for good health. But too much of anything is not healthy. So it is with these essential oils.

Oils rich in essential fatty acids are a good choice for those suffering from arthritis. Essential fatty acids are fragile substances and are easily destroyed in the heating process used to create many of our common vegetable oils.

Flaxseed (Linseed) Oil

One of the best oils is *unrefined, cold-pressed flaxseed (linseed) oil.* It is the only oil which contains both linoleic and linolenic acids, valuable substances in the formation of prostaglandin. Perhaps that is an unfamiliar term to you but prostaglandin are hormones which control many metabolic processes. They affect the cardiovascular system and are present in the lungs, kidneys, pancreas, prostate gland, and even in the brain.

There are more than a dozen important prostaglandin and all are derived from essential fatty acids. If your system is not getting these fatty acids, it cannot produce prostaglandin.

So what does this have to do with your arthritis? A lot! Many experts now see arthritis as a metabolic condition, a dysfunction of the body's metabolism. Arthritis is a drying up and eventually a damaging of the body's joints. Most experts agree, also, that the breakdown process begins with the cartilage of the joints.

With the proper oil, according to many research reports, the cartilage can be lubricated via the nearby joint cavity. The oils, in this manner, are filtered into the cartilage and provide it with extra elasticity, which keeps it from wearing out.

The sensitive part of the process, however, is at the very beginning, when the oil enters your system initially. Once you consume the proper type of oil, for example, unrefined, cold-pressed flaxseed (linseed) oil, the digestive process begins.

Fats or oils that reach the body's duodenum -- a section of the small intestine -- are then emulsified by bile salts and reduced to microscopic droplets. Now the substances are ready for absorption into the blood.

Products, such as amino acids from protein, glucose from carbohydrates, as well as minerals, vitamins and oils, are transferred to finger-like outlets into the wall of the small intestines. All the products, except the oils, pass through the portal vein and enter the liver to be used by the body or to be stored in that organ until needed.

Oils take a different route. In fact, they can go to one of two places. The oils may be collected by the "lymphatic system" and transported around the liver or they can be taken to the portal vein to be delivered to the liver and eventually eliminated.

It is best that the oils by-pass the liver and are transported through the lymphatic system to the joints, where they can be of tremendous value.

How Oils Can Aid Arthritis

To illustrate the changes possible in the body with the use of the right type of oils, listen to the story of G.F., a 63-year-old man. He had suffered from osteoarthritis for several years. It progressively worsened. While aspirin relieved the symptoms temporarily, it bothered his stomach. Mr. F. read about the need for essential fatty acids in the body and the possible link of this deficiency to arthritis.

He included unrefined, cold-pressed flaxseed (linseed) oil in his dietary habits. He took a tablespoon daily, mixed with cottage cheese, tofu or ricotta cheese.

Slowly, he noticed changes. The improvement did not happen overnight -- but he was pleased to see any type of easing in a condition which previously had only been worsening.

Today, his arthritis no longer bothers him. He continues to take unrefined, cold-pressed flaxseed (linseed) oil daily.

The Essential Fatty Acids

The essential fatty acids found in unrefined, cold-pressed flaxseed (linseed) oil are important for overall good health as well as aiding or preventing arthritis. Both linoleic and linolenic acids are vital to life. They also contribute to the prevention of building up of plaque on the arteries.

Another important function of these particular acids is the transportation of oxygen through the body. Every cell requires oxygen. Each organ of the body needs oxygen to function properly. When the membranes surrounding and protecting the cells have this oxygen, harmful bacteria cannot enter.

Essential fatty acids also control chromosomes during cell division and are necessary to the formation of new cell membranes once the cell has divided. Because we know that cancer cells are abnormal cells which grow and perpetuate themselves by division, it is easy to understand why essential fatty acids may be extremely important not only as a preventive measure but also as a form of treatment.

For more information on this topic, see *How to Fight Cancer and Win*, by William L. Fischer, Fischer Publishing, Canfield, Ohio 44406.

Deficiencies May Be Widespread

Many health authorities are only now beginning to realize that deficiencies of essential fatty acids may be more common than previously thought. Research demonstrates that the tissues and blood levels of those suffering from degenerative diseases, such as arthritis, lack the essential fatty acids.

When the diet is lacking in these all-important substances, serious health problems develop. Many "diseases of civilization," such as cancer, heart disease and arthritis are fostered by an excessive intake of saturated fats and chemically-altered fats. These are void of any essential fatty acids.

Saturated fat, hydrogenated and partially hydrogenated oils may have started with the full complement of fatty acids necessary for good health, but the processing system used to prepare them for consumption destroyed any nutritional value they had.

Flaxseed (Linseed) Oil As A Therapeutic Agent

In its unrefined form, flaxseed (linseed) oil contains both linoleic and linolenic acids, better known as

Omega 6 and Omega 3. In fact, of all vegetable oils, flaxseed's percentage of these essential fatty acids is the highest at seventy-two percent. See page 73 to compare the percentage of these essential substances in other oils.

Unrefined, cold-pressed flaxseed (linseed) oil is being used therapeutically by many European physicians who are treating the following conditions:

Conditions	**Benefits**
Arthritis	Exerts a favorable influence
Age-related Complaints	Improves many common deficiencies
Arteriosclerosis	Reduces cholesterol, triglyceride levels
Cancer	Exerts a favorable influence
Eczema	Aids all skin disorders
Bronchial Spasms	Reduces severity
Prostate Gland	Reduces swelling
Intestines	Regulates activity
Stomach Ulcers	Normalizes gastric juices

Conditions	Benefits
Immune Deficiencies	Boost's the body's immune system naturally
Red Blood Corpuscles	Maintains flexibility.

Variety In Using Flaxseed (Linseed) Oil

When used properly, unrefined, cold-pressed flaxseed (linseed) oil has helped people find relief from arthritis-related pain and swelling.

Taking as little as one tablespoonful daily, mixed with cottage cheese, is all many of these people find they need. You may be thinking that this is a boring way to regain your health. But it does not have to be. We have included some recipes to help you vary your intake of unrefined, cold-pressed flaxseed (linseed) oil.

You will be able to find this golden supplement at your local health food store or through select mail order firms which specialize in health products. Just be sure that the brand you buy has not been subjected to the heating process which destroys the essential nutrients.

Value Of Polyunsaturated Oils In Maintaining Good Health

Formation of Prostaglandin Require Both

Linoleic	and	Linolenic Acids
Omega 6		Omega 3

To Prevent

Arthritis	Thrombosis
Cancer	Asthma
Arteriosclerosis	Heart-Related Diseases

If you use these oils, you are supplying your body with:

	Linoleic Acid	**Linolenic Acid**
Flaxseed	14%	58%
Safflower	75%	—
Sunflower	65%	—
Corn	59%	—
Olive	8%	—

Fruity Cottage Cheese A La Flaxseed

1/2 to 1 cup low-fat cottage cheese

1 tablespoon cold-pressed, unrefined flaxseed (linseed) oil

1 handful fresh strawberries (or any other fruit)

Mix cottage cheese and fruit, then add the tablespoon of flaxseed (linseed) oil. Combine well. You may add any type of fruit or vegetable that appeals to you. It is best, however, to use the freshest possible fruits.

Delicious Flaxseed Muesli

Raisins	Grapes	Peaches
Bananas	Pears	Apricots
Apples		

Or any other fresh fruit you prefer.

Mixed nuts (do not use peanuts).

Cream Topping:

3 to 4 oz. low-fat cottage cheese

1 tablespoon honey

1 tablespoon unrefined, cold-pressed flaxseed (linseed) oil

3 tablespoons low-fat milk

In a deep bowl, layer the sliced fresh fruit, alternating with the mixed nuts. Then combine ingredients for the cream topping or mix in an electric mixer or blender. For a creamy consistency, you may need to add a little more low-fat milk.

Spoon the topping over the layered fruit and nuts. You can top off with more chopped nuts, fruits or spices.

Cod Liver Oil

There are a few other oils which may also benefit the arthritis sufferer. Among these is *cod liver oil.*

Recent scientific studies point to the effectiveness of this oil in maintaining good health.

Cod liver oil may be particularly effective for the arthritis sufferer because of its high content of Vitamin D, which is necessary to stimulate calcium absorption. But, for this reason, it should be used very carefully, as an excess of Vitamin D can be toxic to the body.

Experts say that, for maximum effect, you should take a little cod liver oil mixed with orange juice three to four hours after your evening meal. Fresh-squeezed orange juice is best, as it does not contain the preservatives, additives and unnatural sugars of many commercial brands.

Squeeze half an orange and strain the pulp. Place two ounces in a glass along with one tablespoon of cod liver oil. Stir well for thirty to forty-five seconds. You will notice the formation of tiny bubbles. This is fine. Drink immediately.

Do not eat for at least four hours, if you drink this in the evening. You may also take the cod liver oil-orange juice blend in the morning. In this case, you need only wait one and a half to two hours before eating -- the stomach empties more quickly in the morning.

If you wish, you may also take the oil with milk. This may be an excellent choice for those who experience arthritic-related deformities in their joints. According to some specialists, such deformities indicate an allergy to citric acid or fruit sugar.

After several months of using this supplement, you may find that the "drying up" process which has been occurring throughout your body is reversing itself. When you notice an improvement in your dry skin or scalp, you may *gradually* reduce the amount of cod liver oil you take. See page 77 for a list of the symptoms of the "drying out" process.

Eventually, you may only need to take the oil every other day. Let your body be your guide. When you reach this point, stay with the every-other-day dosage for about three months. If you continue to feel good, then you may reduce the frequency to every other week -- which will then be your permanent maintenance dosage.

Those who have diabetes, high blood pressure, related heart disease or gallbladder problems should take the cod liver-orange juice blend only every other day or even twice a week because their bodies cannot assimilate oils as efficiently or as quickly.

If, in addition to arthritis, you also have an ulcer, a nervous condition, dermatitis, eczema, psoriasis, or other skin disorders, you should not use orange juice. Mix your cod liver oil with milk. Very often, these ailments also indicate an allergy to citric acid and fruit sugar.

If you use the orange juice-cod liver oil mixture and experience any discomfort, discontinue use. Take the oil with either milk or alone.

Is Your Body 'Drying Out?"

Dry skin and other areas of dryness on your body may be signals of a lack of proper dietary oils in your diet.

While these symptoms are by no means indications that you currently have arthritis, they may mean that the "drying out" process, which very often proceeds this condition, may be at work in your body. These signals may precede the onset of an arthritic condition by five to ten years.

1) Dry, cracking or inflamed joints.
2) Stiffness upon rising in the morning.
3) Numbing or tingling sensations in the extremities.
4) Cold or clammy hands and legs.
5) Dry skin on different parts of the body.
6) Dandruff.
7) Brittle or splitting fingernails.
8) Etch markings on the teeth.
9) Dry, scaly ears and absence of ear wax.
10) Encrustation in the corners of the eyes.
11) Premature graying of the hair.
12) Wrinkles on the skin.

13) Varicose veins.
14) Bleeding gums.
15) Loss of color change in complexion.

Chapter 4

Herbs And Arthritis Natural Relief

While aspirin is probably the most common over-the-counter pain reliever for arthritis, it is not without its side effects -- especially when used in the large quantities some arthritics need. One of the more common problems encountered by people who use a lot of aspirin is stomach irritation and the possible development of ulcers.

Fortunately, nature has provided us with some alternatives which are less harsh and contain no side effects. These are herbal teas and massages. Herbalists of generations past valued the medicinal qualities of plants and respected their abilities to bring relief of pain -- even the pain of arthritis.

Because each person reacts differently to different remedies, we suggest that you try several herbs to discover the ones which are most effective for you.

The first herbal remedy we present may surprise you. It is the ordinary garden vegetable, the *carrot*. Herbalists suggest those suffering from arthritis receive an abundance of carrots in their diet -- in any form, raw, grated or juiced. This vegetable has been known to diminish the pain of both osteoarthritis and rheumatoid arthritis as well as that of gout.

One of the reasons why carrots may help ease the pain is the wealth of vitamins they contain. We all know they are famous for their high content of Vitamin A, but they also have lots of other nutrients, including the B-Complex vitamins, and Vitamins C, D and E.

Vitamin C, of course, is essential for proper development of connective tissue, which is vital to healthy joints.

It is best to eat carrots raw, because cooking them destroys much of the vitamin content. Try drinking carrot juice in the morning or eat a homemade carrot cereal in place of store-bought, processed cereal.

If you find you can't munch on whole, raw carrots because they are too difficult to bite -- grate them. But don't grate them in advance and store them. The vegetable loses much of its nutrients by sitting. In fact, whatever form you eat the carrot, eat it as fresh as possible.

Moreover, the specific nutrients in carrots stimulate your endocrine glands and protect the nervous system. These same nutrients will also help to provide your body with energy, making you more likely to engage in some type of physical activity. This, too, is a great therapy for arthritics.

The directions for carrot juice and carrot cereal follow.

Carrot Juice

3 large raw carrots

Scrub the carrots well, but do not peel them -- the majority of the vitamins are concentrated near the surface of the vegetable.

Put the carrots in the juicer.

Note: Only make as much juice as you and your family plan to use immediately. Carrot juice loses its nutrient content when exposed to the air for extended periods of time.

Carrot Cereal

1/2 cup oat flakes

1 large carrot, finely grated

milk

Soak the oat flakes in milk overnight. The next morning, finely grate the carrot and add it to the oats.

Warm the mixture slightly and sweeten with honey.

Drinking an herbal tea made of *Club Moss* may help to alleviate the pain of rheumatoid arthritis, according to many who study plants for their medicinal value.

Club Moss is aptly named, for it is a mossy trailing

plant, which has ramblers that reach out and cling to the ground with small, hair-like roots. These ramblers eventually grow into forked branches.

In addition to helping rheumatism, Club Moss also is said to help relieve the often excruciating pain of gout. This natural herbal tea is also reputed to be of benefit to urinary tract and reproductive organs, as well as reducing the inflammation of the testes.

The tea works so well, herbalists say that one cup daily is all a person needs. The directions are listed below.

Club Moss Tea

1 teaspoon Club Moss

1 pint boiling water

Pour the boiling water over the herb and allow it to steep for five minutes. Strain. Sip a cup of the tea each day, one half hour before breakfast.

Another tea which herbalists believe is very effective is *Horsetail.* A cup daily may eliminate the pain of both rheumatism and osteoarthritis, as well as that of gout. In fact, some herbal specialists believe that this herb is so effective against these conditions that it may actually *prevent* their development, when taken regularly. This tea is also excellent if you suffer from water retention or bladder and kidney problems.

The herb, Horsetail, is also known by various other names, including Bottle Brush, Shave Grass, Pewterwort and Dutch Rushes.

The directions for the tea are listed below.

Horsetail Tea

1 heaping teaspoon Horsetail

6 oz. freshly-boiled water

Pour the water over the herb and allow it to steep for four minutes. Strain.

This tea is most effective when taken hot. If you like, you may sweeten it with a little honey.

Because of the potent natural properties of Horsetail Tea, you need only drink one cup daily.

Yarrow is another good herbal choice in natural teas for those suffering with arthritis. Unlike the previous teas, though, you may need to drink more than one cup daily to find relief. In fact, you may want to drink three or four cups every day. And, to increase the effectiveness of Yarrow's natural medicinal powers, you should add a pinch of cayenne pepper to the drink.

Yarrow Tea is also effective for lower back pain and bursitis as well as easing just about any menstrual problem. Some herbalists also recommend this tea for relief of sinus headaches. The directions follow.

Yarrow Tea

1 heaping teaspoon minced Yarrow

6 oz. freshly-boiled water

1 pinch cayenne pepper

Pour the water over the herb and allow it to steep for three to four minutes. Strain. Add cayenne pepper. Do not sweeten.

You may drink up to four cups of this tea daily.

European herbalists recommend their patients take *Stinging Nettle Tea*, with some *Swedish Bitters* added. They suggest that a person begin to drink about half a cup of this mixture prior to their meals and another half cup after eating.

Swedish Bitters, an herbal blend, may be found in your local health food store. If your store does not carry it, there are several mail order firms that do.

The directions for making Stinging Nettle Tea follow.

Stinging Nettle Tea

1 heaping teaspoon Stinging Nettle

6 oz. freshly-boiled water

Pour the water over the herb and allow it to steep for three minutes. Strain. Add two teaspoons Swedish Bitters. Sip hot.

Drink about one half cup before each meal. Drink another half cup following the meal.

Another herbal tea recommended to arthritics consists of a blend of plants, carefully chosen for their healing properties. It is suggested that you drink four cups of this Herbal Blend Tea daily. The instructions follow.

Herbal Blend Tea

1 pinch Chamomile	2 pinches Violet
1 pinch Lavender	2 pinches Rosemary
2 pinches Sage	2 pints freshly-boiled water

Pour the water over the herbs and allow to steep for three to five minutes. Strain. Sip hot. You may drink up to four cups daily.

Dandelion Tea, when taken daily, may act as a detoxifying agent, cleansing the bloodstream of impurities which, according to many physicians, is a contributing cause of arthritis. For best results, drink a cup of this tea one half hour before breakfast and a half hour after breakfast daily. The directions are provided below.

Dandelion Tea

2 heaping tablespoons dried dandelion root

or

1 tablespoon fresh dandelion root

2 cups cold water

Chop dandelion root into fine pieces and soak it in water overnight. The following day, bring the mixture to a boil. Strain.

Drink twice daily -- a half hour before breakfast and a half hour after breakfast.

Feverfew

Feverfew has been considered a very valuable herb in the treatment of many ailments, including arthritis. This herb, which bears a flower resembling a daisy, is considered a most effective remedy for migraine headaches and perhaps is best known for its ability to relieve this pain. But Feverfew is also very useful as a natural treatment for arthritic pain. The plant has become so popular that you can find it in capsule form in just about any health food store.

Some people believe that the herb actually helps reduce the inflammation associated with arthritis. Recent evidence also indicates that it may even help prevent the process which leads to the inflammation. Medical research is still being conducted on this remarkable plant.

Karen P., 62, originally began taking Feverfew capsules for her persistent migraine headaches. She soon discovered what she considered a delightful bonus -- an improvement in her arthritis.

"I realized my joints didn't ache as they used to," she said. "At first I didn't connect it with my taking Feverfew. But then I learned it really was the capsules which were helping me ease my pain. Now I feel as if I have a new lease on life. For the past couple of years, I have been taking Feverfew and I've been doing work my arthritis would not allow me to do before.

Henry J., 66, used Feverfew for his arthritis. "I began taking the capsules because my wife read it might help my condition. It had gotten so painful I couldn't even work in the garden anymore. My garden, at one time, was my pride and joy."

Henry said that he was very skeptical about the herb. "After all," he conceded, "I had visited every doctor in town. If this herb really did work, why didn't they tell me about it?"

But his wife persisted and Henry figured that Feverfew couldn't do any damage. Within a remarkably short period of time, he said, "I noticed a distinct improvement in my condition. Before very long, I was back in my garden -- with a minimum amount of pain.

"Feverfew is wonderful. I wish someone would have told me about it years ago."

Herbalists say that Feverfew is one of the more powerful of natural remedies and, for this reason, should not be used by pregnant women, breast-feeding mothers, babies or children.

Because Feverfew has only recently been available commercially, many people grow their own plants and then eat the leaves to find relief. The taste of this plant is very strong and bitter. Many times people will eat the leaves as part of a sandwich, in an attempt to disguise the bitterness of the leaves.

If you decide to grow your own, there are a few precautions you should know. You should grow a minimum of three plants -- two to set seeds for new sprouts and the third to harvest for your treatments. The plant which you use as your supply of Feverfew should not be allowed to flower.

If you eat the fresh plant, you may experience some side effects, the most common being a soreness in the mouth. This problem may also affect the tongue and perhaps cause swelling of the lips. A small percentage of people have noticed a rash when eating the plant fresh.

There are several brands of Feverfew but, when purchasing this herbal aid, take caution to choose only the kind made from all natural ingredients for the best possible results. You should be able to find these products at health food stores and through reputable mail-order outlets.

Herbal Massages

Massages are always a great aid in helping to

relieve the stiffness of muscles and joints, whether the cause be arthritis or overuse. When you can add some herbal oils or ointments to the massage, you have increased its therapeutic value. There are several herbs which are particularly effective as massage aids.

One of the best is *Marjoram Oil.* The warming effects of this herbal aid, when used in gentle rubbing action, help to relieve the pain and aching joints and help to relax stiff muscles. Apply the oil and massage gently into the affected area when needed. Directions for making Marjoram Oil follow.

Marjoram Massage Oil

Marjoram

Cold-pressed olive oil

Glass jar

Lightly crush enough of the herb to fill the jar halfway. Do not use a plastic container. Then fill the jar with olive oil. Cap tightly and place the bottle in a warm place. Allow it to sit for three weeks.

At the end of that period, strain and use the herb-soaked oil as a massage aid.

Another herbal oil, reputed to help ease the pain and stiffness of joints is *St. John's Wort.* It is also an excellent natural treatment for sprained and pulled muscles. The directions for making the oil follow.

St. John's Wort Massage Oil

Fresh St. John's Wort flowers and leaves

Olive oil

Glass jar

Place a quantity of the herb in the bottle until it is about three quarters loosely filled. The amount of herbs needed will depend upon the size of the glass jar used.

Then fill the jar with cold-pressed olive oil. Cap tightly and place in a warm place for approximately three to four weeks. You will know when the mixture is ready to strain, because it turns red.

After you have strained it, you may use the oil as a massage aid. It should be stored away from the light. St. John's Wort oil keeps its potency for up to two years.

We have already mentioned the Stinging Nettle herb as a useful treatment when taken as a tea. It is also a very good treatment when used as a massage. However, you need not create an oil to have an effective herbal massage aid in this plant. It is quite helpful when rubbed into the body as a tea. Herbalists say that massaging the body with Stinging Nettle Tea may also improve your circulation.

This herbal infusion may be added to your bath to ease the pain and stiffness of arthritis. The instructions for the tea are located on page 84. For these purposes, omit the Swedish Bitters called for in the recipe.

Poultices To Relieve Pain

Two herbs, used in poultice form and applied to the joints, may help relieve the pain of arthritis.

Comfrey is the first of these. Herbalists have long touted this plant as aiding in the healing of all types of bruises and even in speeding the healing of fractured bones.

A Comfrey poultice may also be useful to those who suffer with varicose veins or gout. In fact, we have included the guidelines on making a Comfrey poultice in our chapter on gout, because it has proven so effective for this problem. See page 143.

A poultice made from the herb Horsetail is also said to provide relief for this condition. It is especially effective when allowed to remain on the affected area overnight. Directions for making this herbal remedy follow.

Horsetail Poultice

2 handfuls Horsetail

Place the herb in a colander and sit it over a saucepan of boiling water. Cover the colander tightly to keep the steam from escaping. Allow it to steam until the herb is soft and hot.

Wrap the steamed herb in a white cloth and apply it to the affected area. Fasten it securely.

You may want to wrap this with another cloth to keep the moist heat from escaping.

Devil's Claw

With the name *Devil's Claw* you would hardly expect this African herb to be a blessing to arthritis sufferers but, indeed, it is.

Scientific testing has proven it remarkably effective in reducing the pain and swelling of arthritis in rats and increasing the mobility of their joints.

According to studies, Devil's Claw is effective because it is a diuretic and a cleanser. Current research indicates that the herb reduces the inflammation by extracting the superfluous fluid from the affected joint areas. This allows the connective tissue to function normally and act as a barrier against toxins.

The testimonies of people worldwide indicate that relief may be available for you.

A nine-year-old girl, Karen, was helped by this herb. She had a severe case of rheumatoid arthritis which kept her in constant pain. Her parents had sought all the best doctors and tried everything the medical community had to offer -- but Karen continued in daily pain.

Finally, her parents heard about Devil's Claw and tried it. Within two months, the herb reduced Karen's pain considerably.

Today, Karen is able to enjoy life as other children do. She swims regularly and is an enthusiastic, and very good, gymnast.

Bertha M., 74, also suffered from an extreme case of arthritis, which she developed in her early forties. For over thirty years, she endured the pain.

Her daughter then learned about Devil's Claw bark. Bertha took a four-week treatment of these tablets daily. She described her improvement as miraculous. Her daughter is elated, saying, "Now my mother is baking cakes and cooking meals and looking after herself once again."

The Devil's Claw plant has an extremely long root system because, as a native of the Kalahari Desert in Africa, it must survive up to ten months of drought conditions each year. It is this root which is the valuable portion of the herb.

Some people have tried Devil's Claw Root Tea, but this is a very bitter drink and few people can tolerate the taste. However, this potent medicinal root is now available in tablet form. There are several different brands on the market and some of these are not made from the herb's root, which is the only portion of the plant possessing medicinal qualities. Be careful when purchasing this product, therefore, and insist on a brand which is made only from the root. Your local health food store should be able to assist you. Devil's Claw is also available through select mail-order houses.

Natural Treatment And Prevention Guide

Herbal Remedies

Herbs	**How It Works**
Carrot	Taken in any form, may reduce pain.
Dandelion	Chewing stems or taken as a tea, may help reduce the pain and swelling of joints.
Devil's Claw	May help reduce symptoms of arthritis. Available in capsule form.
Feverfew	May help reduce pain and swelling and increase mobility of joints. Available in capsule form.
Horsetail Tea	May act as a natural pain reliever.
Marjoram Oil	Rubbed into sore, stiff joints, may provide relief.

Chapter 5

Arthritis And Exercise: A Beneficial Combination

Is it possible to exercise your arthritis away? Well, not quite. But physical activity is an essential component of any arthritis self-help program. It is a less expensive alternative to harsh medications and, while the results may not be immediate, they almost always do occur. In some instances, a regular exercise program, practiced faithfully, may actually eliminate the need for surgery.

On certain days when it feels as if every bone in your body is aching, you are probably not very enthusiastic about exercise. And, indeed, doctors say that, on those days, rest is the perfect treatment.

But the person suffering from this disease needs to find a healthy balance between rest and exercise. It is imperative, if you have not already developed an exercise program, that you do so carefully. Do not be hesitant about contacting your physician and seeking his or her help. Keep in mind, when outlining your goals, your other possible health problems. If you have a heart condition or atherosclerosis, you should obviously ease into activities very slowly.

Walking is an excellent exercise to start. Begin with just ten minutes daily; less if you have difficulties.

The added benefit of walking outdoors is your exposure to sunlight, which stimulates your body's production of Vitamin D. This nutrient is essential for proper calcium absorption, an important consideration for arthritics.

Exercises performed in water are also a good choice for the arthritis sufferer. The water reduces the amount of pressure upon the joints while the exercises are being performed. Some YMCA's hold water exercise classes specifically for those with arthritic-like conditions. Check with your local Y to find out if they conduct such sessions.

There are exercises, additionally, that have been designed for arthritics to perform in the privacy of their homes in the bathtub. These activities have been developed by Nancy Kadler, a nationally-registered Occupational Therapist, who has more than twenty years of professional experience both in hospitals and private clinics.

We would like to share some of these with you because we believe they may help ease the pain of your arthritis and increase your mobility. For more of these bathtub exercises, consult the book *Bathtub Exercises for Arthritis and Back Pain*, by Nancy Kadler and Judy Jetter (E.P. Dutton, N.Y. 1986).

Those who are in a severely weakened physical state should limit their initial exercise regimen to only two or three repetitions of the exercises and perform only a small portion of those provided. As you gain strength, you may gradually increase the number of repetitions, as well as adding more exercises.

Tips To Start

The water temperature of the bathtub should be comfortable, allowing the sore, tight muscles and joints to relax. Temperatures between 85 degrees to not more than 90 degrees Fahrenheit are usually best. But do not spend more than forty-five minutes exercising in these temperatures.

The number of times you perform these exercises is your choice and the decision should be based upon your level of strength and the severity of your arthritis. You may want to start out with ten repetitions of the exercises. It is probably best to start with three repetitions of each activity and slowly increase the number as you go along.

You will not achieve immediate results, so do not overdo it in hopes of hurrying improvement. These exercises are not designed for that type of progress.

All instructions are written with the understanding that you are sitting in your bathtub. If you are using a hot tub instead, you may need to modify the directions slightly.

Feet Synchronization

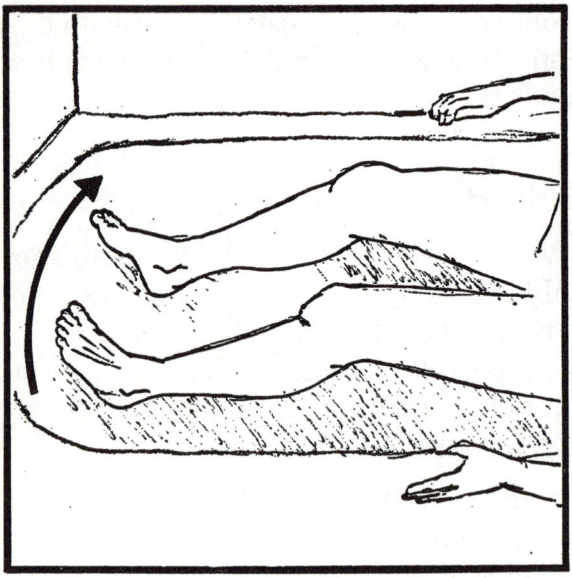

Facing forward, with your legs extended, turn both feet to the right, as far as possible without discomfort. The outside edge of your right foot and the inside edge of your left foot should be resting on or near the bottom of the tub.

Rotate both feet in the opposite direction. Now, the outside edge of your left foot and the inside edge of your right foot will be resting on or near the tub's bottom.

Repeat these rotations once.

Next, point each foot toward the other (so the toes are near each other). Then, point the feet in the opposite direction, so the closest part of the feet are the heels. Repeat.

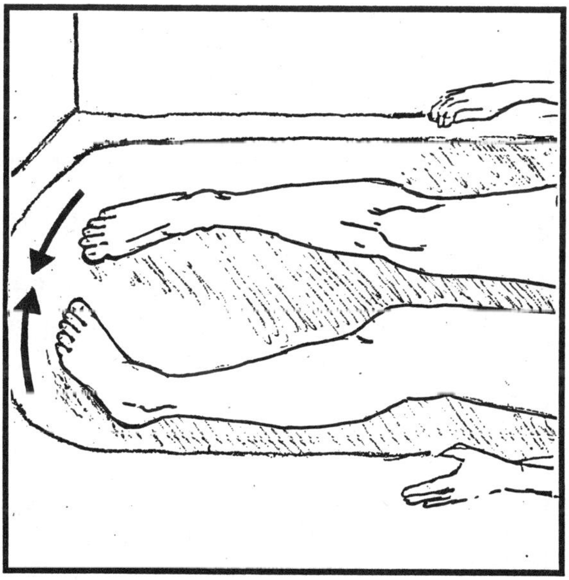

Finger Swings

Sit with your knees apart. Submerge your hands in the tub water, keeping your palms down and your elbows straight. Bend your wrists, allowing your fingers to drop until the back of your hands face the floor. Your fingers are parallel with the tub's bottom.

If you cannot bend your wrists this much, bend them as far as you can *comfortably*.

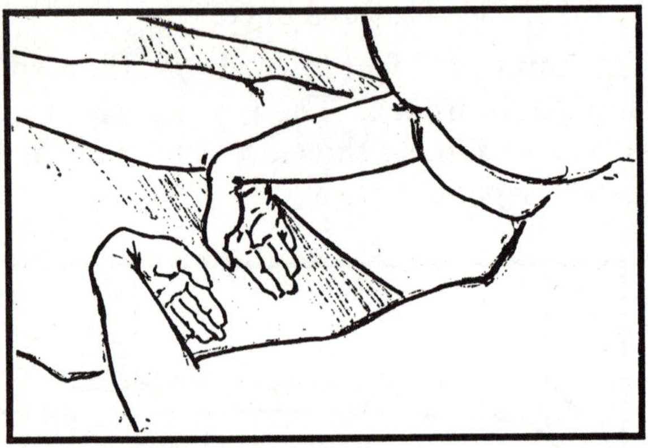

Keep your wrists at the same depth in the water, while you slowly raise your fingers as they point upward as high as is comfortable. Do not force your fingers. Hold this position for a count of three. You should feel some tension through your wrist and forearm. Repeat.

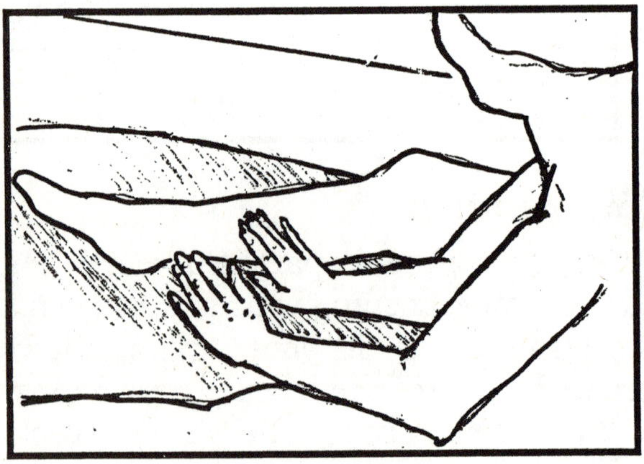

Foot Stretches

Sit comfortably in the tub and spread your knees slightly. Point your toes toward the ceiling. If you can, point them toward your face. Hold for a count of three. You should feel the muscles in your calves tighten.

Slowly lower your toes until they point away from you. Hold for a count of three.

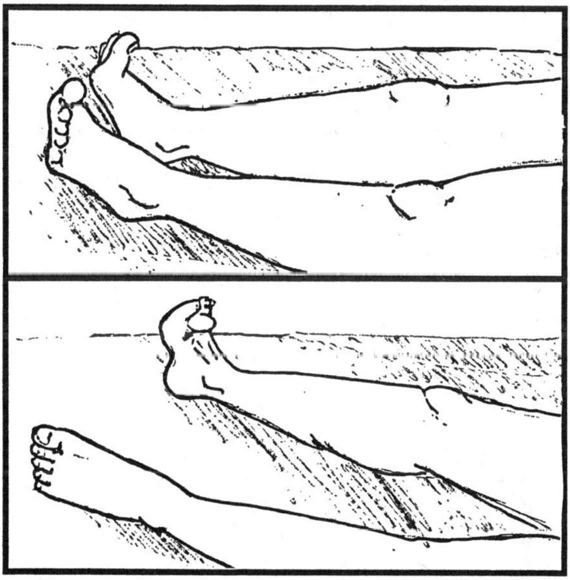

If you wish, also perform a variation of this by pointing your left foot away from you and your right foot toward you (or toward the ceiling, depending upon your mobility). Hold for a count of three. Reverse the feet positions.

Swing and Stretch

This exercise works the feet as in the *Foot Stretches* and the wrists and fingers as described in the *Finger Swings.*

Submerge your hands in the water, between your knees. Point both your hands and your feet up and then point them down. (Your feet should be pointing away from your body and towards the tub.) Hold each position for a count of three.

Try any variety of this, pointing your hands down and your feet up or one foot up and the other away from you, while alternating the same pattern with your hands. Each time, hold the position for a count of three.

Toe Holds

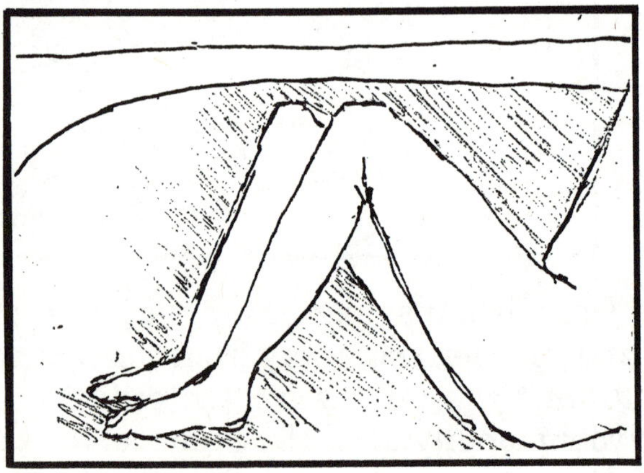

Sitting in the tub, bend your knees so your feet are

lying flat on the tub floor. Raise your big toes as high as possible. Your other toes will automatically move. Do not worry about that.

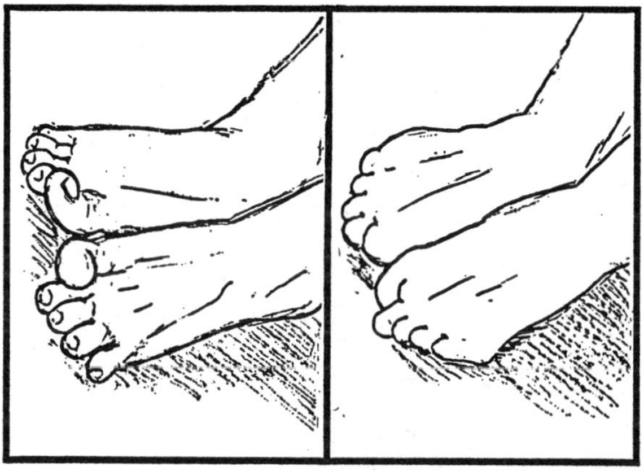

Next, curl your big toe and hold it as close to the balls of your feet as possible. Do not lift your feet any higher than absolutely necessary. Again, your other toes will also move.

Thumb Cross

With your knees spread comfortably, submerge your outstretched arms between them. Your fingers should be straight and your palms up.

Cross each thumb over the palm, until it reaches the base of the little finger. If you cannot stretch it this far, do not worry and do not force it. In this case, cross your thumb as far as it will go over the palm comfortably. Try not to cup your hands.

Return your thumbs to their original position. Cross the thumbs over the palms again, this time only as far as the base of the ring finger (or as far as it will go comfortably).

Repeat this for the other two fingers as well.

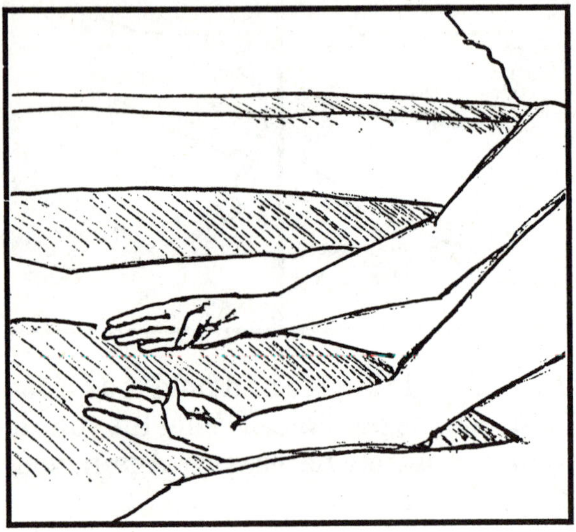

Deep Breathing Exercises

Deep breathing exercises are very beneficial to arthritis sufferers. They help to relieve tension, improve circulation, promote the elimination of toxins from the body, as well as aid in the digestion of food. Additionally, such exercises expand the chest muscles and provide your body with increased oxygen which helps in strengthening and rebuilding your health.

The following are two exercises which should be performed regularly:

Lie flat on your back on a hard surface, preferably the floor. With your mouth closed, slowly inhale deeply through both nostrils. Hold this breath as long as possible. Exhale slowly.

Repeat this five times initially. Gradually increase the number you perform to ten. If you cannot perform this five times, do as many as possible and slowly work up to five.

Next, block the left nostril with your finger and perform the deep breathing exercise as explained above. Do this two times.

Repeat the process but this time block the right nostril. Repeat twice.

Stretching Exercises

The following are several exercises, all based on gentle stretching. As with the previous activities, stretch only as long as it is comfortable. The exercise provided below should not promote pain when performed correctly. If you feel pain as you do them, stop. Try the activity again but do not stretch as far this time.

Do all of these exercises slowly. Do not hurry through them and do not try to do them all in your first session in hopes of speeding relief. Unfortunately, our bodies do not react that way to physical activity.

Standing Stretch

Stand with your feet apart. Bend your legs slightly. Clasp your hands behind your back. Very slowly, bend forward from the waist while raising your arms behind your back.

Go only as far as is comfortable. When you have stretched as far as your body will allow, hold the position for a count of five. Then slowly reverse the process to return to your original position.

Repeat this exercise once.

Seated Stretch

Sit on the floor. Extend your legs and put your knees together. Exhale, then slowly stretch your upper body forward, sliding your hands downward. Your goal is to touch your ankles. The first few times you perform this exercise you may not be able to reach the ankles. Just go as far as is comfortable. If you feel pain, stop. Hold for a count of five. Slowly return to your original position.

Perform this stretch three times.

Knee Pulls

Lie on your back with your feet extended. Place your hands at your sides. Slowly pull your right leg towards your chest as far as is comfortable without pain. Grasp the leg with both arms and hold this position for a count of five. Lower your leg to the floor.

Repeat the process with your left leg. Perform this activity three times, if possible.

Next pull both of your legs as close to your chest as possible without pain. Lock your arms around your knees. Hold this for a count of five. If you can keep this position for a count of fifteen without pain, you may do so.

Repeat this once.

Hip Rotators

Lie on your back with your arms at your sides as in the knee pulls. Place your palms down. Pull your knees toward your chest. With your hands on the floor used as supports, rotate your hips and legs to the left as far as possible. Your goal is to have your legs touch the floor. You may not be able to achieve this with the first attempt. Do not become discouraged.

Your shoulders and back should remain flat against the floor during this stretch.

Reverse your position slowly, bringing your legs towards your chest and then gently placing them back on the floor.

Repeat the procedure and rotate your hips to the right.

Perform this exercise two times, if possible.

Neck Stretches

Sitting straight, bend your neck to the left as far as you can comfortably. You are trying to reach your shoulder.

Next bend your neck to the right, again, go only as far as is comfortable, but aim for the shoulder.

Repeat this five times.

Next, rotate your neck slowly as far as you can comfortably to one side, then to the other. Repeat this five times, if possible. If not, do as many as you can without pain and slowly work up to five.

Rebounding

You would think that the rebounder was designed with arthritics in mind, so beneficial is it to those suffering with this condition. The rebounder is a revolutionary approach to exercise that is easy on the joints, yet provides maximum benefits. Few other exercise programs can make that claim.

Rebounding is probably the most efficient form of exercise ever devised. It involves gentle movement upon a personal-sized rebounder. There are even hand rails provided for easy mounting and dismounting as well as security while rebounding.

Ethel M. had suffered from arthritis for many years, but in the past several months her condition had steadily declined. This not only worried her but it also upset her husband, Carl, quite a bit.

One day Carl came home with a large box. Ethel asked what was in it. "You'll see," replied her husband.

Carl quickly assembled the rebounder and showed

it to his wife. "This is for you," he said proudly. "It's going to help some of that pain of yours."

Ethel just laughed. She could barely move from room to room; did he really expect her to actually exercise?

He stepped onto the rebounder and showed her how to "bounce" on it. Then he quickly added, "But, Ethel, you don't even have to do that much if you're not up to it. Just stand on there and get used to it."

She was a bit apprehensive but it seemed to mean so much to Carl that she tried it. She got onto the rebounder, carefully holding the handrail. She bounced very gently, never letting go of the rails. She was not on the rebounder for very long, just long enough for about 25 bounces.

The following day, she tried the rebounder again. This time she did a little more. By the end of the week, she noticed a slight improvement. This encouraged her and she continued. By the end of the month, Ethel found it much easier to get around and her pain was lessened considerably.

Soon this 68-year-old woman was singing as she cleaned her house and whistling as she crocheted -- a hobby she thought she would never again enjoy.

"I thought my husband was crazy when he brought the rebounder home for me to use," she said. "I never in a million years expected to use that thing. And I never thought my arthritis would improve. I am so grateful to Carl."

Exercise: The Key To Staying Young

Medical science has discovered the key to staying youthful. Exercise. A 60-year-old who exercised regularly all his life can be as fit as a younger person who gets little or no exercise, science is now determining.

Read the stories of those rare individuals who have lived to be 100 years or more. What is the common thread running through them all: exercise in some form. It may be that they did physical labor of some type, such as working in the fields, every day of their lives.

In fact, many of these individuals had "silent heart disease." But, because their hearts were very healthy, they were not fatally affected. The same health problem, though, in a weaker heart, would have been fatal.

"But," you say, "I'm already affected by arthritis. I'm not going to live to be 100 -- and it's probably too late for me to start improving my health."

It is never too late!

You can, indeed, experience the benefits of exercise even if you have a severe case of arthritis. While such strenuous activities as jogging and tennis may be beyond you, rebounding is within your reach. Because this marvelous exercise is available to you, don't think that it is any less beneficial than other activities. In fact, NASA evaluated rebounding recently and determined it to be 68 percent more effective than jogging, which has been touted as one of the best forms of physical activity available.

And perhaps the best advantage to rebounding is its convenience. You can perform it whenever and wherever you want, in the privacy of your own home or office. And there is no need to postpone your exercise because of rain or snow.

When the rebounder is not in use, it folds up quickly and easily to fit in a closet or under the bed.

How Does Rebounding Work?

How can mere gentle bouncing on a rebounder give your body such fantastic results? This exercise, unlike many others, stimulates every single cell in your body simultaneously! Rebounding uses the natural forces of gravity to work its wonders.

We all know that gravity was first recognized as a force by Isaac Newton who, legend contends, was hit on the head with an apple falling from a tree.

Gravity is literally pulling on all objects of the atmosphere. Therefore, we are all subjected to this force; even our cells are influenced. But the only way this law can be used to develop strength is by opposing it in some way.

Let's take the exercise of push-ups as an example. When you perform this activity, your body interacts with gravity in the following ways:

1) Opposing gravity with the muscles of your arms.
2) Accelerating the top of your body at the beginning of the push.
3) Decelerating only the top of your body as your chest touches the floor.

Similarly, the same forces are at work when you rebound. When you stand motionless on the rebounder, every cell in your body opposes gravity. If you were to take your bathroom scale and place it on the rebounder under your feet, it would register your weight.

However, this changes as you begin to bounce. At the bottom of the bounce, the needle on the scale would register more and it would show the combined forces of gravity plus the deceleration which your body experiences in its downward thrust and acceleration when the expanded springs of the rebounder contract and force your body back up.

Even without allowing your feet to leave the mat, the gravitational forces would increase by almost twenty-five percent.

This means that every cell in your body is directly affected by the increase. Bouncing on a rebounder stresses your cells approximately one hundred times in a minute. This repetition will force the cells to adapt to this greater gravitational force and thus become stronger.

Making Rebounding A Part Of Your Life

It takes only a little bit of discipline to make rebounding an integral part of your life. It is so easy and takes such a small amount of time to notice results, you will find it an easy habit to keep. Here are some suggestions to make rebounding part of your daily lifestyle.

1) Establish a specific area for rebounding.

Select an area or room of your house or office where you will perform this exercise. Try not to vary this.

2) Keep the rebounder available in this special place.

When you do this, all you need to do is jump on. If it is put away after each use, you will have to decide if you want to take it out now or later. And, if it is always out, you can "steal" an extra minute or so on it anytime you wish. If it is always set up, the rebounder is always available to every member of the family, regardless of his or her busy personal schedule.

3) To achieve maximum benefits, rebound within the first three to five minutes after you get out of bed.

Not only will this help you wake up, but rebounding early stimulates your cells to burn more calories all day long. Your cells will work more efficiently.

Exercising first thing in the morning also helps decrease your dependence on your morning cup of coffee.

4) Increase your time on the rebounder only when your body is ready.

While the fashionable phrase in exercise is "no pain, no gain," that does not hold true here. Do not exercise until you are sore. Slowly work up to ten minutes daily. At first you may only be able to stay on the rebounder for thirty seconds or so -- don't worry. That is enough until your body gets into shape. Physical exercise experts estimate that ten minutes of rebounding is the approximate equivalent of thirty minutes of jogging. Give yourself a pat on the back for what time -- no matter how short -- you are spending on the rebounder. Positive reinforcement will encourage you to continue.

5) Provide variety in your exercise routine.

One day you may rebound to some upbeat music, other days you might decide to exercise while you are watching the news or your favorite television program. Rebounding while watching television brings more benefits than snacking in front of the set.

Test The Results Of Rebounding For Yourself

Try this simple "test" at home to demonstrate the remarkable effect rebounding has on every single cell of your body.

1) Sit on the floor, legs extended out before you. Place your hands on your lap.

2) Have a friend place a hand on your chest and push your upper body backwards. Do not use your hands to support yourself. Keep them on your lap, but do try to resist this force.

You will find you cannot keep your body in an upright position.

3) Now jump on the rebounder and jog in place for three minutes.

4) Return to the first position of sitting on the floor. With legs extended and hands on your lap, once again ask the same person to push you backwards. Resist, just as you did before.

Because every cell in your body responded to the increased gravitational forces of rebounding, you will find you have little trouble resisting the person this time.

For more information on the availability of this revolutionary new device, contact *The Rebound Fitness Society*, whose address is provided below.

The Rebound Fitness Society

P.O. Box 116

Canfield, Ohio 44406

216/ 533-5673

Remarkable Effects On The Immune System

Rebounding, recent studies show, may even increase the functioning of your immune system. The same gravitational forces we have been talking about with this activity can be graphically illustrated through space travel. Swiss scientists have discovered that cells weakened by a loss of gravity are also less strong to withstand diseases.

During space travel, astronauts become weightless. These Swiss researchers have shown that this state also produced a corresponding inhibition in the immune system. Following a careful examination of the white blood cells of both American and Soviet space travellers, the researchers subjected the weakened cells to a greater gravitational force.

The immune system responded to this by becoming stronger and more active.

Rebounding subjects the entire body to additional gravitation, stimulating the body's immune system defenses. You may find that, after using the rebounder, not only is your arthritis less bothersome but you no longer develop the colds and flu as you did before.

Chapter 6

Hidden Secrets To Overcoming Arthritis

Dr. Hanne Kramb, N.D., a highly respected naturopathic physician and founder of the world-famous Hanne Kramb Clinic in Germany, experienced remarkable results with the use of new, natural, homeopathic tablets, used in conjunction with two very special herbal teas.

This unique treatment has already helped thousand of Europeans beat the pain and agony of arthritis. Called *Rheumapac,* the tablets are a precisely-blended combination of fifteen homeopathic medicines. When used along with the teas, *G-26* and *G-27*, it proves to be extremely effective. Arthritis sufferers are asked to drink a good quantity of hot water with the tablets.

Beneficial effects are noticed within a short period of time. Symptoms which have been with some people for years are eased with as little as several doses of Rheumapac and the teas.

"I'm so very pleased to be able to help people," Dr. Kramb said. "until very recently, I could do little as a doctor to help my patients. It made me feel helpless. But now, it is very heartening to know that this remedy, which is natural and very safe, can help those with arthritis and arthritic-like conditions.

"Moreover, I'm pleased because my patients no longer have to contend with the very often powerful adverse side effects of arthritis drugs. When the tablets are used as directed, a good deal of hot water is taken with it, and the teas are consumed, a marvelous change is noticed in the health of the person."

Hans D. visited Dr. Kramb, telling her he had tried everything for his painful rheumatoid arthritis. Nothing seemed to help. In fact, some of the strong medications physicians gave him only made his condition worse, he said. Would Dr. Kramb have anything at all that might help, he wondered?

The naturopathic physician told him to take Rheumapac as well as the teas, G-26 and G-27, as she directed. "I think Hans was skeptical at first," the doctor said. "he wasn't expecting a 'prescription' for tea. I told him to come back in several weeks. When he returned, I hardly recognized him. He was a changed man.

"His aches, he told me, had disappeared, and he once again looked forward to getting out of bed each morning. He smiled and laughed his way through our office visit. It was a real pleasure chatting with him.

What a contrast to his first visit, where he sat practically motionless and seldom spoke beyond answering questions."

This new, natural breakthrough treatment is now available in the United States. Rheumapac and the therapeutic teas, G-26 and G-27, may be just the remedy that will help ease your arthritis condition. These products are all natural and extremely safe to take. There are no adverse side effects and they work in a relatively short period of time.

These remarkable products will be available shortly through better health food stores and select mail-order outlets specializing in health-related products.

The Great Grape Diet

If someone told you that he cured himself of arthritis by eating nothing but grapes, you might not believe him. But do not dismiss his account until you have learned all the facts.

The facts seem to indicate that, indeed, people are improving their health dramatically, ridding their bodies of toxins which cause not only arthritis and rheumatism, but also ulcers, various skin disorders, migraine headaches, even serious conditions such as inflammation of the kidneys, using this diet.

These, though, are only a few of the ailments which can be alleviated with the Great Grape Diet, a simple and extremely effective, short-term eating plan based on the healing properties of the grape -- a perfectly balanced fruit.

Balance is the key word to this plan. By eating nothing but grapes for about one month, the body is restored to a natural healthy balance which nature intended it to be. This is something that cannot be accomplished through the use of antibiotics since these synthetic chemicals can kill off the healthy organisms of your system as they destroy the illness-producing ones.

The grape treatment requires living for a limited period of time on fresh, ripe, sweet grapes which are well washed. The length of time is obviously determined by your state of health at the start of the program, the type of illness you have and the progress you make while on the treatment.

No other food may be eaten and you may only drink water which has been boiled. Hot water is taken when you feel nauseous; cold when you are thirsty.

You should not smoke under any circumstances while on this program, nor should you take any drugs. (Smoking is also discouraged once you have regained your health.)

Expect a loss of weight from anywhere between three to eight pounds per week, the first several weeks you are on the Great Grape Diet. This, of course, is not a cause for concern, but is a necessary component of the plan. However, once all the poisons are dissolved and eliminated from your system, your weight will stabilize and shortly thereafter even increase -- without adding any other food to your diet.

It is highly recommended that you consult a nutrition-minded doctor before you begin this treatment.

Nutritive Power

The glucose and fructose of the grape -- natural sugars -- are responsible for the potent nutritional value of the grape. No other fruit contains a higher percentage of these sugars, which are easily assimilated by the body without the aid of insulin. This fact greatly enhances the renewal of tissues, giving new life and vitality to exhausted and debilitated organisms.

And since the sugars found in the grape burn rapidly, the body is given an extra amount of energy which, in turn, saves the protein reserve, an important part of the biological economy of the human system.

Grapes contain a wealth of vitamins which are essential to good health -- and are especially important for the arthritic -- including Vitamin C, A, and several of the B-Complex. This fruit is also a great source of organic acids, such as Malic, Citric and Tartaric, which are the basis of mineral salts. Mineral salts, such as potassium sodium, calcium, phosphorus and iron are essential to the health of the human body. They not only contribute to an alkalizing effect but also promote a natural diuretic action extremely beneficial to the body.

How Long A Diet? How Many Grapes?

Many people go on the Great Grape Diet for about thirty days. It takes at least three weeks until you notice a distinct improvement in your health. While this may seem a long time, it must be kept in mind that your ailment did not develop overnight. Illnesses are the result of years of abuse in the form of poor eating habits. It is unrealistic, then, to expect a fast cure.

In fact, the therapy should not be any shorter than four weeks for the treatment of a chronic illness. Do not make the mistake of stopping the therapy prematurely merely because you feel great. While your body may feel better, that does not ensure that the toxins are all eliminated. If they are still in your system, and you quit the diet too soon, you may experience a recurrence of the ailment.

While on the diet, do not be afraid to eat a lot of grapes. Some people report that they eat as much as five pounds on their first day alone. Find the right amount that will satisfy you without over-filling you. But do remember, do not eat anything but the grapes. If you eat any other food (other than boiled water), you will achieve no results at all.

You may notice that, while on the diet, you develop

a headache the first week or so. This is normal and only means that the elimination of the toxins is causing your bloodstream a little irritation. Do not allow the headaches to stop your program.

Some people also notice changes in the color of their urine and stool. Again, don't become upset, as this is one of the mechanisms your body uses to eliminate poisons.

Once the bloodstream is thoroughly cleansed, all diseases will have been removed from your body. To keep your health good, refrain from alcohol and cigarettes while eating a diet of naturally healthy foods.

The Healing Qualities Of Clay

Clay has been used to cure many ailments for centuries. While the modern technology of today has overshadowed its natural healing properties, clay once again is becoming a popular and effective way to help ease arthritis.

In fact, a combination of clay and herbs can have lasting effects upon this condition. The clay is mixed into a paste and a hot herbal infusion is added for a poultice. This is applied to the affected part of the body, for a "double action" of natural, potent healing.

However, if you decide to try this method, be extremely careful on what problems, other than arthritis, you use it. Do not apply it to a boil, in an attempt to collect the pus and draw it to a head.

Clay poultices may be applied either hot or cold, depending upon the time of the year and the individual's sensitivities. It may be more comfortable to apply a hot poultice during the winter months than the summer ones. Similarly, a cold poultice may be easier to wear during the hot summer months.

For a small clay poultice, mix one tablespoon of clay (for source information, see the Appendix on page 217) with an herb infusion (see Chapter 4 for the best herbs to use on arthritis) and mix this into a thin paste. Evenly spread the paste about a quarter of an inch thick on the affected part of the body.

As the clay dries, it will become brittle and hard which may make removal of the poultice uncomfortable for those with sensitive skin. If you have this condition, you should try to keep the clay moist. Mixing a little St. John's Wort Oil with the poultice accomplishes this nicely. Applying the poultice at night, moreover, is the least obtrusive method.

For chronic cases of rheumatism and arthritis, alternating the clay poultice with one made of pulped white cabbage produces the most beneficial effects. This method also has been recommended in some cases of cancerous growths.

A cabbage poultice is probably the easiest type to make. Since the vegetable leaves contain a gentle-acting, healing effect, there is no fear of them coming in direct contact with the skin, as with some more stringent leaves. Heat the white cabbage leaves after you have pulped them. This can even be done with an ordinary clothes iron. Apply the poultice to the affected area and wrap it with a piece of linen.

Do not keep the poultice on for longer than five minutes. A series of short applications with frequent breaks will do your joints more good than a single, long, uninterrupted one.

Stimulate Circulation

As in the case of most ailments, arthritis and rheumatism are aggravated, if not partially caused by, poor circulation. Stimulating your circulatory system, therefore, will greatly aid your arthritic condition.

This can be done by simply taking hot and cold showers and vigorously rubbing the skin twice a day.

Similarly, a twice-weekly bath with Epsom Salts is also recommended. Or you may consider massaging your painful joints with baking powder, while they are submerged in water.

Put The Freeze On Arthritis

An excellent way to relieve your body of arthritic pain is through ice therapy. This is a simple but effective form of treatment and can be carried out with just an ordinary ice pack, if necessary.

Fill an ice pack with up to ten ice cubes and apply it below or above the joint that hurts. Do not put it directly on the joint. Wrap a towel around the pack and let is sit snugly for about a half an hour. At first, you will obviously feel the cold but this changes to a warming sensation, which later will be numb. Repeat this several times throughout the day as needed.

If your hands or feet are afflicted with arthritis, a contrast bath is an excellent remedy. You will need two basins. Fill the first with ice water and the other with water that is comfortably hot. Do not make the water so hot that you cannot place your hands or feet into it.

Start with the hot water and soak the affected limbs for ten minutes. Then place the limbs into the cold water for only one minute. Continue this pattern for thirty minutes. Not only will you notice that your pain has eased, but you will discover that your fingers or toes are more mobile. For maximum benefit, you should end the session with the one minute in the cold bath.

While this form of therapy has no side effects for the vast majority of people, those with diabetes, Raynaud's Syndrome, and collagen and blood conditions should use hydrotherapy and ice therapy only under a physician's supervision.

Walking Barefoot

This remedy may seem too simple -- and too enjoyable -- but many people have found relief with it. Walk barefoot in the early morning grass while it is still wet with dew. This grounds the static electricity in your body and helps to regenerate your energy. After your early morning barefoot stroll, vigorously dry your feet with a rough towel and put on a pair of shoes immediately.

If you live in the middle of a city and this remedy is impossible for you to carry out, then have a friend massage your feet daily with olive oil blended well with ten drops of pine oil.

The Circulizer System

Mary P. thought nothing could help her arthritis pain. It bothered her both day and night. While everyone told her just to live with it, that advice was difficult to follow. Living with pain is not easy.

Her daughter, naturally concerned about her mother's health, read everything she could find about the ways to ease the pain of this terrible joint condition. She discovered a unique foot bath, called *The Circulizer System*. After Mary had used it just several times, her pain had eased considerably. Mary was amazed at how much better she felt. Her daughter was grateful that the Circulizer had worked. Mary is now performing tasks that she thought she would never do again.

The Circulizer System is a footbath into which you place specially developed herbal blends. The warming action on your feet will help improve the circulation of your blood throughout the body and, after several uses, begin to alleviate many health problems.

Joe R. also suffered from arthritis. In addition to pain, he had lost a lot of mobility in his arms. This, naturally, limited the activities he could enjoy. Not accepting his physical condition, Joe searched for a means of improving his state of health. He finally found The Circulizer. After several warm, herbal water treatments of The Circulizer, Joe felt much better.

"To say that my pain no longer bothers me would be an understatement," Joe explained. "It felt wonderful not to be bothered by the aches. But it felt even better to be able to move my arms once again. I hadn't experienced that joy in years."

The Circulizer Explained

How does this Circulizer Footbath work? Its remarkable abilities are based on a simple phenomenon known as *Dastre-Moratsche* or the consensual reaction. This reaction is much simpler to illustrate than to explain. A person goes for a walk on a cold, wintry day. He accidentally walks over some ice which he had assumed was fully frozen. It was not.

The ice breaks and he steps into extremely cold water. His boots and socks are soaked, as well as his feet. This causes a drastic lowering of the temperature of the sensitive thermal receptors on the soles of his feet. He soon develops a serious head cold. Even though his head was not involved in the accident, the person's nose and sinus cavities are affected by the change in temperature of his feet. Measurements show that the temperature of the mucous membranes of the velum, oral cavity and outer auditory canals drop when the feet are cold.

Using this principle, you can, with The Circulizer, gradually raise the temperature of these body parts and thus aid your well being. The Circulizer's benefits begin at the feet by first expanding the tiny capillaries in the soles. As the temperature slowly rises, the deep-seated, larger arterioles and the large blood vessels of the feet expand.

In a relatively short period of time, all the blood vessels of the feet are expanded as far as possible and the beneficial effects of the herbs soon travel throughout the body.

Revolutionary Approach

Extensive testing has proven The Circulizer to be a revolutionary approach to the many health problems related to, or complicated by, poor circulation. Many specialists agree that arthritis is a health problem that is caused by, or aggravated by, poor circulation. In many cases, the toxins which produce the swelling and the pain cannot be eliminated because the blood is not flowing properly throughout the body.

Poor circulation may be more prevalent than we suspect. In our society, fewer people than ever before are obtaining the exercise they need to stimulate proper blood flow. Sitting at a desk for eight to ten hours a day leaves little time for physical activities.

But the herbal footbath can compensate for this by helping to increase your circulation. And the footbath can be used in the privacy of your own home. The footbath is a self-contained unit which is filled with water and a special blend of herbs. It is gradually warmed not only to aid the circulatory system, but also to bring out the maximum medicinal benefits of the herbs.

Scientific study has now confirmed the beneficial qualities of herbs. When used with the controlled temperature increase, they are greatly enhanced.

Arthritis is not the only condition which benefits from The Circulizer. Any other health problem stemming from impaired blood flow can be improved with the use of the footbath, including, angina, asthma, migraine headaches, intermittent claudication, high cholesterol, diabetes, high triglyceride levels, dizziness, arteriosclerosis, osteoporosis, high and low blood pressure, heart arrhythmia, lupus erythematosus, prostate problems, psoriasis, eczema, insomnia and much, much more.

Mrs. M.N. is extremely pleased with the results she received using this miraculous footbath. "I am convinced of the good effect of the herbal bath. I no longer suffer from the rheumatism that made me miserable for more than twenty years."

Flush Away Toxins

When used with precisely-blended herbs, the controlled temperature footbath system helps to flush the toxins out of the body while improving circulation. Modern medicine is only now appreciating the fact that the skin is the largest eliminative organ of the body. Many impurities are excreted through the pores of the skin, carried outside along with perspiration, which controls the temperature of the body.

Toxins play a large role in causing all types of arthritis as well as the pain and immobility associated with the disease. Employing The Circulizer, with changes in your diet, as outlined in Chapter 2, should go a long way to keeping your body free of toxins. The benefits will appear sooner than you think and you will feel better than you have in years.

Relieve Constipation -- Naturally

No one likes to talk about it but constipation is a condition which many arthritics share. Studies have been done recently which confirm that those people who suffer with arthritis need a longer period of time to properly eliminate toxins and other materials from their bodies.

Previously, there was little a person could do for this situation, aside from taking often harsh, chemically-based laxatives. These commercial products, found by the truckload in the stores, very often do more harm than good. Instead of cleansing the system of the toxins, these products may actually add more toxins to the body.

Now there is a natural alternative. *Naturalax* is a name given to a recipe from Europe that provides a gentle way to ease constipation and help cleanse the system. Naturalax, which you can make at home, offers you relief quickly and without danger to your body. It is a unique and wonderful option that allows you to take control of your health.

Many of the laxatives found on your drug store shelf contain a derivative of senna which can be harmful if taken for a prolonged period of time. These senna derivatives erode the intestinal floor if not used sparingly.

On the other hand, Naturalax, used by many people in Europe, is extremely safe for all people. It carries none of the harsh side effects found in many of the products that are frequently used today. And you may take the Naturalax, that you have prepared yourself, without fear of hurting your system.

Naturalax exercises the colon and makes the digestive system work smoothly because its high content of mucous causes peristalsis. It's low in calories and can be taken by diabetics. One to four days of use is needed to see results.

Naturalax

makes 1,000 grams (about 2 lbs.)

30 grams yeast powder or yeast flakes

20 grams wheat germ

100 grams whole blonde psyllium seed (not husks)

350 grams whole flaxseed

150 grams whey powder

350 grams mustard seed

Take one to two tablespoons with tea, milk, coffee or a glass of water each morning before breakfast. MUST BE SWALLOWED, NOT CHEWED, FOR BEST EFFECT. For thorough cleansing, drink at least 8 glasses of water each day.

Or you may want to try a Naturalax Drink that is enjoyed by many health-conscious Europeans. To make the Drink, mix one to two tablespoons of Naturalax in a glass of warm water. Add one to two teaspoons of honey and sprinkle liberally with whey powder. Drink the liquids, then eat the rest by spoonfuls.

Lawrence K. had suffered from constipation for several years. He was not quite sure what was causing it as he watched his diet very closely. Despite this care, he found himself needing a laxative to ease the problem.

But Lawrence was also concerned about what these products were doing to his body. He felt sure that the items he took to help his condition ultimately were doing more harm than good.

A friend told him about Naturalax and the relief he

had obtained from it. Lawrence gave it a try. He was impressed with the speed and gentleness of this all-natural product and soon felt a general increase in his overall well being. Today, he is not bothered by constipation.

Chapter 7
Gout and Bursitis

David P. was awakened early one Sunday morning by a pain in his foot. He discovered that the big toe on his left foot was extremely swollen and red.

The night before, this 55-year-old businessman had indulged in a victory celebration of the closing of a major deal for his firm. He had enjoyed a very elegant and rich dinner at one of the best French restaurants in town. He ate pate, filet mignon with brandied cream sauce, as well as three glasses of wine and chocolate mousse and liqueur for dessert.

But now, less than twenty-four hours later, the pain was too much for him to endure. He was not even able to bear the weight of the bedsheet on his toe. Obviously, he could not put a shoe on and walking was out of the question.

Monday morning, David hobbled to a rheumatologist, an expert in arthritic conditions. The doctor confirmed, through blood tests, that David had developed a case of *gout*.

David's condition grew better with treatment. The doctor prescribed indomethacin (Indocin) but David learned a valuable lesson -- the hard way. He discovered the very real connection between his diet and his health.

Gout is a relative of arthritis and, in fact, is also called gouty arthritis. Historically, it has been considered a disease of the affluent and has long been associated with a diet rich in meats -- especially organ meats -- and alcohol. The stereotypical gout sufferer, in many people's minds, is a portly, middle-aged man.

Medical experts now say that, indeed, an excessively high intake of organ meats and alcohol does increase the body's uric acid level, which may precipitate a case of gout. The consumption of these foods was once limited to the wealthy of society, which is how the condition became associated with affluence.

Today, these rich foods are common fare for many people, regardless of their economic status -- a fact reflected by the incidence of gout among even those who do not have a lot of money.

Diagnosing Gout

Physicians make the diagnosis of gout upon the presence of deposits of fine, needle-like crystals of uric acid somewhere in the body. This disease is the most well known form of crystal-induced joint inflammation.

Gout occurs when excessive amounts of uric acid accumulate in the body and crystals collect in the connective tissues. These uric acid crystals are most commonly found in the joints. Over several years, the crystals coalesce to form larger collections, called *tophi*. These are often visible, appearing as nodules just below the surface of the skin and usually found in the elbows and on the hands.

The Course Of An Attack

An acute attack of gout strikes quite suddenly and peaks very quickly. Not infrequently, the first pain will occur in the middle of the night and awaken the person. It usually begins as an infection of the big toe, which appears hot, tender and inflamed. Sometimes other joints of the feet will be involved, or even the ankle or wrist.

This initial attack is extremely painful. Mild acute attacks of gout subside just as quickly as they developed, but tend to recur regularly. Severe attacks, though, may last for days or even weeks.

Most people experience their second attack of gout within six months to two years of the first one. In others, it will take five to ten years for another to develop. These delayed second attacks are more common in those who failed to seek treatment for the initial bout. The recurrences are usually more severe and last longer than the first. They may also affect more joints than the first bout did.

Eventually, chronic gout sets in. This is when the tophi begin to develop.

Kidneys And Gout

Damage from gout is not limited to your joints; the kidneys, in rare instance, may also be harmed by the uric acid. Just as the tophi are visible in various joints of the chronic gout sufferer, they may also be forming on the lining of the kidneys.

In fact, kidney damage is probably a more threatening, long-term consequence of the disease than is joint damage. Kidneys affected by uric acid pose a threat to the person because the organ may fail to eliminate waste products properly or the condition may contribute to high blood pressure. In some cases, kidney failure and ultimately death may follow.

Where Does Uric Acid Come From?

It is true that much of the uric acid content of the body originates in our diet -- especially in the form of meat and alcohol. However, some is also produced by the body itself, through the constant creation and dying off of the body's cells. Biologists call this process *cell turnover* -- new cells being manufactured to replace the old ones.

In certain blood conditions and skin diseases, though, the amount of cell turnover is increased, and so is the amount of uric acid. Psoriasis is a disease with excessive cell turnover. Many times, people with psoriasis also develop gout. Polycythemia, the presence of too many red blood cells in the blood, is another disease which produces an excessive amount of uric acid.

Gout And Aspirin Do Not Mix

If you suffer from gout, you should avoid taking aspirin. This may seem strange. After all, gout is a form of arthritis and aspirin is the best known drug for arthritis.

But *acetylsalicylic acid*, the technical term for aspirin, is one of several drugs which are slightly acid and may slow the rate at which your body eliminates uric acid. There are other drugs, such as diuretics, which help the body get rid of excessive fluid, which may also impede uric acid elimination.

If you develop gout and are taking other medication, consult the physician who prescribed it and explain your new health problem to him or her. He, or she, may be able to provide you with an alternative, but equally effective, drug.

Diet Modification

The best way to eliminate uric acid from your system is through a non-citrus, alkaline fast of about three to four days. These fasts may be repeated often, over a six-month period, to ensure all the acid leaves the body.

A diet high in alkaline fluids helps to keep the uric

acid from crystallizing, while drinking plenty of liquids aid in its elimination. The best juices for the fast are non-citrus fruit juices, cherry juice, celery and parsley juices, vegetable juice and potassium broth.

Between fasting periods, you should follow a diet low in uric acid, purine and fat. Also abstain from alcohol during this time. Try to make three-quarters of your diet raw foods, especially concentrating on non-starchy vegetables. Those most recommended by naturopathic physicians are cabbage, kale, alfalfa sprouts, carrots, celery and parsley. Also include in this diet plenty of bing cherries, bananas and strawberries.

The ideal situation is to follow this pattern of eating, eliminating all refined carbohydrates and protein for five days between your first and second liquid fasts.

If you find this too difficult to do, then introduce low-purine foods to your system slowly. The best sources of these are raw goat's milk and goat's yogurt, poached eggs, brown rice millet, corn bread and low-fat cheeses. However, keep the bulk of your diet composed of the green vegetables listed above.

Long Term Modification

Once you have eliminated the uric acid from your system, it would be wise to follow a sound diet which is low in purine, the substance which encourages crystalline formation. Also, getting in the habit of drinking plenty of liquids will help encourage regular uric acid elimination.

Below are lists of food categories gout sufferers should be aware of for long-term avoidance of the disease. The first category contains low-purine foods, which you may freely add to your diet. The second group contains a moderate amount of purine. While eating foods from this list, on occasion, will not do you harm, do not use these foods as the main components of your new eating patterns or you will develop more gout. The third list outlines the foods which are high in purine and should be eliminated from your diet.

Low-Purine Foods

These foods may be eaten freely by gout sufferers.

Millet	Goat's Yogurt	Nuts
Rice	Eggs (Poached)	Cornbread
Goat's Milk	Green Vegetables	Fruit

Foods With Moderate Purine Content

These foods may be eaten in small quantities by those prone to gout.

Bran	Shellfish	Fish
Asparagus	Mushrooms	Beans
Lentils	Cauliflower	Peas
Chicken	Whole Wheat	Spinach

Food With High Purine Content

Those prone to gout should avoid these foods.

Anchovies	Mackerel	Sardines
Yeast	Meat Broth	Herring
Roe	Oatmeal	Spices
Scallops	Organ Meats	

Garlic As A Remedy For Gout

In Russia, garlic is issued for more than just seasoning. It is also used as a remedy for relieving the pain of gout. The method the Russians use is to take two cloves of garlic and mince them very fine. Place this in a glass of water and drink the mixture down very fast. No chewing of the garlic is required.

An Americanized version of this remedy puts the minced garlic into a glass of cherry juice. If you use this method, be sure to buy juice which contains no preservatives or added sugars. You can find it in your local health food store.

Herbal Remedies

There are several natural, herbal remedies which have been known to help relieve the pain of gout.

The most well-known of these is *Comfrey*, a plant which grows in clumps and has large, fuzzy, dark green leaves. Comfrey has pale pink bell-shaped flowers.

Herbalists recommend using this herb as a poultice applied to the big toe (or any other joint bothered by the condition). Apply the poultice to your toe as needed to ease the pain. The instructions for the herbal compress follow.

Comfrey Poultice

2 handfuls fresh comfrey root

1/4 cup water

Wash and clean the root. Chop it finely and place in an oven, set on low heat, until the root is dried. Grind into a meal. While it is still warm, mix with enough water to make a paste. Add a few drops of cold-pressed olive oil to the paste.

Spread the herbal paste onto a clean, white cloth and apply it to the toe. Snugly fasten the poultice.

You may use the poultice as needed. Keep it as warm as possible. Change if it cools.

Two herbal teas may help eliminate toxins from your body and, in the process, ease your pain. The first is *Club Moss*, a trailing plant with mossy-like surface that puts forth ramblers which cling to the ground.

In addition to helping gout, Club Moss tea is also reputed to help chronic constipation, urinary tract infections and problems with the liver and the kidneys.

The instructions for this tea may be found on page 82, in the chapter on herbs and arthritis.

Cherries

We mentioned earlier the fact that you might want to include cherries as part of your diet modification program in hopes of avoiding recurring gout attacks. This fruit has long been noted, in folk medicine and by early twentieth century physicians, to help alleviate the pain of the disease.

It was not uncommon in the early 1900s for physicians in the United States to "prescribe" the eating of cherries to their patients who came to them with a case of gout.

In fact, in 1950, Ludwig Blau, Ph.D., wrote an article in the journal *Texas Reports on Biology and Medicine*, explaining cherries' role in curing him of gout. Blau was not a typical gout sufferer. He had developed the disease so bad that he was confined to a wheelchair. But, he said, eating six to eight cherries daily eventually controlled and cured this health problem. As long as he continued to eat this fruit, the gout stayed away.

Other people contend that you should begin by eating fifteen to twenty-five cherries the first few days on this regimen, then gradually reduce it to ten daily.

Naturopathic physicians include cherries and

cherry juice into the diets of their patients complaining of gout because they say it neutralizes the uric acid.

Gout And The Beer Drinker

If you drink beer regularly and drink lots of it, you may be setting yourself up for an attack of gout. Beer is one of those foods high in purine, which the body converts to uric acid. A recent study in England showed that beer drinking was the most crucial difference between those who developed the disease and those who were free from it.

Forty-one percent of the gout sufferers in the study drank more than seven cans of beer daily. Only seventeen percent of the healthy men consumed that quantity.

Pseudogout

Uric acid is not the only crystalline substance capable of producing pain in your joints. *Pseudogout,* also called *Chondrocalcinosis,* is the result of deposits of crystals composed of calcium salts which accumulate in the joints.

This condition, more often than not, attacks older people and usually develops gradually, in contrast to gout's sudden, acute episodes.

Pseudogout also differs from its cousin, gout, in

that it usually affects the larger joints and most often the knee. It may also occur, but usually not as frequently, in the wrist, elbow, shoulder, hip or spine.

An episode of pseudogout may be triggered by an injury or surgery or, in some instance, both. Unlike gout, diet plays no role in its emergence. It may develop, though, as a result of another disease, such as diabetes, Wilson's disease or hyperparathyroidism.

Unfortunately, scientists have yet to identify the metabolic malfunction which is responsible for the development of pseudogout.

The symptoms of this condition include inflammation of the joint, accompanied by warmth or stiffness. Pain is also noticed in the area.

In some cases, the skin covering the affected joint will be red. Once these symptoms are noticed, the episode will continue for a prolonged period of time, not reaching its peak for twelve to thirty-six hours.

Since the cause of the deposits is still unknown, so is an effective treatment. Some physicians are able to relieve pain and swelling by draining off a portion of the fluid from the sore joint, which will eliminate some of the crystals. But that treatment does not prevent a recurrence of the disease.

Bursitis

Bursitis is an inflammation of the bursa, a small sac located between tendons and bones, around certain joints. The bursae may also be found between layers of muscle. Their purpose is to provide a cushioning barrier to these areas, otherwise susceptible to tissue damage. The movement involved in these areas creates friction; the bursae help to reduce that.

Examples of bursitis include tennis elbow and housemaid's knee. The shoulder, though, is probably the most common site for this inflammation and it is called *subdeltoid* when it occurs here.

Symptoms of this disease include painful swelling of the joint and restriction of movement. The area affected may be tender to the touch and appear red. Muscular weakness may also be present and the person may even experience a fever.

The condition has numerous causes, including the result of arthritis or gout. But there are two major causes of bursitis -- direct trauma and microtrauma.

Direct trauma refers to an injury. An injury to the shoulder, for example, causes the bursa to swell, which produces general swelling in the area and restricted movement of the joint.

Bursitis caused in this manner heals fairly quickly if the affected part of the body is well rested. This is an example of acute bursitis. Rest is extremely important. If the joint is forced to perform too soon following the injury, the chances are greatly increased that you may develop chronic bursitis, which is just as the name implies; it stays with you many years.

The second common cause of bursitis is microtrauma or repeated uses of the area. A carpenter, for example, may sustain microtrauma to his shoulder due to his frequent use of a hammer. Or he may develop bursitis in his elbow due to the frequent use of a screwdriver. The same principle is involved when you develop tennis elbow.

While none of these motions asks the body to perform something it is incapable of doing, the problem occurs following a prolonged period of use. Eventually, this may cause irritation and inflammation of the bursa.

In chronic bursitis, the wall of the bursa may become thickened which may prompt muscular weakness.

Vitamin C May Help

If you suffer from chronic bursitis, you should examine your nutritional status. You may be deficient in Vitamin C. Doctors now know that high levels of Vitamin C aid in the protection of connective tissues and may actually help guard against such injuries. It is possible that your body may be able to sustain a higher amount of microtrauma without injury to the bursa, if it had higher reserves of Vitamin C.

If you suspect that this is your problem, augment

your diet with Vitamin C rich foods (see the chart below). A healthy diet is the best way to receive your nutrients. If that is not possible, though, do not hesitate to take vitamin supplements. When choosing a tablet, be sure to notice if the formula contains Vitamin C with Bioflavonoid. This substance is found naturally in all foods containing Vitamin C, but it is not found in all supplement formulas.

While you will be able to find a good quality Vitamin C formula in your local health food store, do not overlook the reputable mail order firms which offer this particular and very potent Vitamin C supplement. Many of these firms provide the consumer with excellent quality products at reasonable prices.

Best Natural Sources of Vitamin C

You probably know that ascorbic acid, better known as Vitamin C, may help prevent colds. But what you might not realize is this nutrient's amazing ability to help protect connective tissue, which is exactly the type found in the bursa.

Doctors and researchers alike now theorize that bursitis may be avoided if the body has a healthy supply of this nutrient. This would help keep the connective tissue in top working order and make it more resistant to microtrauma, or repeated use.

If you perform an activity or are in an occupation which requires repeated use of your arm or other parts of your body, you may wish to add more Vitamin C to your diet.

Below are listed some of the best natural sources of Vitamin C:

Cabbage	Potatoes	Parsley
Kale	Citrus Fruits	Watercress
Black Currants	Green Peppers	Broccoli
Brussel Sprouts		

Rest Your Joint -- Then Exercise It

Try to use the joint affected by bursitis as little as possible for the first forty-eight hours. You may even want to wear it in a sling to keep the limb from being used.

During this period apply cold compresses (see page 125) as often as every three hours.

But, after this period, once the pain and swelling are beginning to subside, physicians encourage gentle exercise. This not only speeds the healing process, but also reduces the chances of adhesions forming, which may ultimately limit the mobility of the joint.

Your exercise program should begin with passive mobilization, the movement of the injured joint with the aid of another person. Perform this type of activity at least two times per day, but no more than six. This exercises the joint to its full range of motion without the use of the patient's muscle. There are now machines made for this purpose which have been extremely successful in contributing to the healing of soft tissues and joints.

The next step in the healing process is exercising the joints alone through activities which require no muscle movement. Two are particularly good, the Easy Arm Swing and the Toe Touch. Both are described below. Do these once a day.

Easy Arm Swing

Bend from the waist and allow your arms to swing freely. Then, very gently, swing your arms from the front to back and then from side to side several times. Do not use your shoulder muscles.

Next, swing your arms in small circles. Gradually increase the diameter of the circles each day of the program. Again, be very gentle in your swings. Circle not more than five times.

The Toe Touch

Simply bend forward at your waist and touch your toes at least five times. You may gradually increase the number each day of the program.

Muscle-Assisted Exercise

The term "muscle-assisted" refers to the fact that some voluntary movement of your muscles is required for the activity's performance. Once you can perform the Easy Arm Swing and the Toe Touch without significant pain, you may begin following this set of exercises.

The Wall Climber

Stand about one foot from a wall, facing it. Place your hands on the wall at a level which is comfortable. Waist level is recommended. Very slowly, move your hands up the wall in much the manner of a spider -- by pulling your fingers forward and back.

Stop as soon as you reach the height where the pain gets worse.

Do this exercise five times daily.

You may want to mark the level you reach on the wall. Then you can try to exceed that on the following days. Your goal is to be able to raise your arms overhead.

Erect Arm Swing

Standing upright, gently swing your arms across your body several times.

As your exercise program continues, you should be able to gradually swing large motions front to back, until you can make a full circle painlessly.

Tying The Apron

If you have an apron, put it on. Then tie it in back. Do this several times. It works just the right muscles. If you do not have an apron, you can go through the motions of the tying of a knot in back of you, waist high.

Picking Your Pocket

Another simple movement which works the muscles is the act of removing a wallet from back pants pocket. Perform this several times a day.

Hydrotherapy For Bursitis

To help relieve the pain and swelling of *acute bursitis*, many physicians recommend a cold compress be placed on the affected area. The simplest way to make a compress is with a wash cloth, saturated with very cold water and the excess water wrung out.

Leave the cold cloth on for about twenty minutes -- replacing it or re-wetting it with cold water during that time if necessary.

Repeat this process several times a day. You may even leave the compress on overnight if you wish.

For *chronic bursitis*, many physicians recommend a hot compress be applied in the same fashion and the same length of time as the cold one.

Poultices

Applying poultices to the joint affected with bursitis may help ease the pain. The two herbs recommended for use in this manner are *Comfrey Root* and *Coltsfoot* teas.

Additionally, another plant is highly recommended for use as a poultice even though we consider it a vegetable and not an herb. It is *cabbage*. Naturopathic physicians and herbalists alike recommend the leaves of this plant as a natural way to draw out bursitis pain.

Making a poultice is simple. If you are using cabbage or coltsfoot leaves, simply spread the fresh leaves evenly on a white cloth large enough to cover the area affected.

Next, crush the leaves. You may do this with a wooden spoon, or, if it is a larger poultice, you may use a rolling pin. This crushes the plant's juices onto the cloth and improves the effectiveness of the compress.

Apply this cloth to the body and then cover it with a woolen over-wrap, if possible. This may be kept on overnight.

If you choose a comfrey root poultice, you will need to dry the root first. Simply place the root, after you have cleaned it and chopped it very fine, into an oven set no higher than 100 degrees. Once the moisture has been drawn out of them, the roots should be ground into a meal and then mixed with enough hot water to make a paste. To this, add two or three drops of cold-pressed olive oil.

Spread this mixture evenly onto the white cloth and fasten it to the joint.

Herbal Massages

Massages always seem to ease the soreness of aches and pains and a brisk massage of the painful joint with the herb *Speedwell* is an excellent addition to your overall care of bursitis, herbalists say.

You will need to use a tincture of the herb, though, and it requires two weeks to soak in spirits. If you are plagued by chronic bursitis, you can make the tincture and store it. For an acute case, though, this method may be impractical.

Speedwell is a slender plant, with clusters of pale blue flowers growing from its hair stem. The leaves are small and toothed, appearing almost like a silvery green and are grouped in pairs.

To prepare the tincture, take two handfuls of the herb, very finely minced. You should use all the parts of the plant except its roots. (Use flowers, leaves and stems.) Put this in a quart glass jar. Fill the jar with spirits -- vodka is fine. Cover it.

Allow to remain undisturbed in a warm place for two weeks. After this time period, you may use it as a massage aid.

Bunions -- A Form Of Bursitis

According to many podiatrists, a bunion is one of the most distressing problems your toe can encounter. Those of us who have suffered through them heartily agree with the experts. It is not only ugly, but it is extremely painful and it makes wearing shoes unbearable. Ant, to top it off, bunions come in pairs.

A bunion is a form of bursitis, indicative of degenerative changes which are taking place in the bone. Most of the time, this condition is accompanied by a deviation of the big toe, called *Hallux Abducto Valgus*. This is the medical jargon meaning "turning away." The bunion may be causing the toe to push inward against the other digits, creating a hammertoe.

Women develop bunions more often than men, for reasons not yet known. Some people have blamed the female's love of stylish, and often uncomfortable, shoes. But this alone does not account for the high incidence of bunions. One possible explanation is that women have a lighter bone structure and are thus more susceptible to this foot condition.

Self Help For Bunions

The best immediate care you can give your bunion is *ice*. Apply ice packs to the affected toe for fifteen minutes. Do this three or four times daily and the inflammation should be reduced.

Also reduce the pressure on the area by wearing a

very wide shoe, open-toed sandals or even a tennis shoe with a hole cut out to accommodate the bunion.

You may also make your own bunion pad by cutting foam rubber into the shape of a doughnut and applying it to the affected area.

Apple Cider Vinegar For Bunions

If you are prone to chronic inflammation of the toe, try soaking your toe in an apple cider vinegar and water mixture. Use one cup of apple cider vinegar to a gallon of warm water. Allow your foot to soak for fifteen minutes.

Gout

Guide To Natural Treatment And Prevention

As a form of arthritis, Gout may be effectively treated with the natural remedies suggested for arthritis.

Natural Remedies	How It Works
Diet	Eat foods low in uric acid content, avoiding organ meats and alcohol. Two-thirds of your diet should consist of non-starchy vegetables.

Bursitis
Guide To Natural Treatment And Prevention

Vitamins	**How It Works**
Vitamin C	Essential for the health and proper functioning of connective tissue.

Other Natural Remedies	
Hydrotherapy	Cold compresses on affected area for twenty minutes in cases of acute bursitis. Hot compresses on area for twenty minutes for chronic bursitis.

Chapter 8

Very Special Supplements To Regain Health

Can a supplement originally developed to strengthen the heart be of any value to those who suffer from arthritis?

Yes, it just might be — a fact more arthritics are discovering daily.

The supplement is a formula developed for his own use by Dr. Jacobus Rinse, born and educated in Holland with a doctorate in physical chemistry. Dr. Rinse was told, following a heart attack at age 51, that he had only ten years to live and only if he restricted all physical activity and continued on medications.

Years of serious research resulted in his creation of a potent natural formula which not only helps the heart but also the body's bones. Today, Dr. Rinse is an active 92-year-old man, a far cry from the terrible prediction of his cardiologist some forty years ago.

Created expressly for the benefit of the body's heart, the added bonus of this remarkable formula is its ability to relieve other health conditions as well, including arthritis.

The formula contains a host of essential vitamins and minerals important to good health, but usually missing from the many processed foods we eat daily.

Elizabeth J. began taking the formula for her heart and was delighted when she noticed an improvement in her arthritis. Today, this 65-year-old woman says, "I am totally free of the arthritic pain which has bothered me for the past ten years."

Perhaps the secret to this formula's success is the way it appears to improve the body's circulation. While this food supplement cleans the blood vessels and arteries which may be partially clogged by atherosclerotic plaque, the results very often affect arthritis and other health conditions.

Joyce P. of Des Moines, Iowa, has suffered from poor circulation. She had trouble even walking up and down a flight of stairs without huffing and puffing. She began taking the Dutch chemist's formula to improve her circulatory system. "Within a few weeks of using the supplement," she said enthusiastically, "I noticed I could run upstairs without breathing heavy."

What she did not expect was the lessening of her pain and swelling from arthritis. Her knees were particularly affected. She says, " All this has stopped now. What a miracle."

The Formula Explained

The ingredients chosen for Dr. Rinse's formula are specially designed to provide your body with the extra vitamins and minerals essential to good health. A quick look at the individual components of this supplement and it is easy to see why arthritis sufferers are favorably affected.

Lecithin

Included for its ability to counteract excess cholesterol in the cardiovascular system, lecithin is a boon to those afflicted with arthritis. In Greek, this word means "egg yolk" and, indeed, that is the best source of lecithin. Liver is also another excellent natural source. Lecithin also contains two B vitamins, choline and inositol.

A deficiency of lecithin may be related to the aging process since this substance is needed in every cell of the body. Lecithin is one of the essential building blocks for the repair of weak cells and organs. Moreover, it helps the body assimilate Vitamins A and E.

Lecithin is particularly important for arthritics because it helps to cleanse the liver and to keep fats in solution.

Brewer's Yeast

This ingredient contains an abundance of the B vitamins, especially pantothenic acid, which is extremely important for the joints. Recent studies indicate that this nutrient may be able to reduce the pain and stiffness of arthritis.

Bone Meal

Bone meal is an especially good source of calcium, which many nutritionists agree arthritics need. Other minerals found in bone meal are zinc, copper, iodine, cobalt, iron, manganese and sulphur. More and more doctors are recommending bone meal supplements to their patients suffering from this joint condition.

Vitamin E

The formula developed by Dr. Rinse includes Vitamin E. This nutrient, researchers have only recently discovered, reduces the swelling and pain of arthritis.

Wheat Germ

This is the primary source of natural Vitamin E and, of all the cereals, wheat germ contributes the most to good health. Additionally, it is an excellent source of the B vitamins.

Vitamin C

Also known as ascorbic acid, this nutrient supplies a type of "cementing" substance that binds cells together in the blood vessels. A deficiency of Vitamin C causes capillary fragility, which may produce such symptoms as spongy and bleeding gums. Moreover, ascorbic acid is vital to the maintenance of the body's connective tissue. Large amounts of aspirin, often taken by arthritis patients, deplete the body's reserves of this vitamin. Vitamin C, additionally, enhances the effectiveness of any medication.

Sunflower Oil

This is a great source of linoleic acid which is also essential for the health of the body's joints. The proper oils keep the joints well lubricated and less susceptible to developing arthritic conditions. If you decide to make the Dr. Rinse Formula yourself, the directions are given below.

Dr. Rinse's Formula

7 tablespoons Lecithin granules
6 tablespoons raw wheat germ
6 tablespoons debittered Brewer's Yeast
(powder or flakes)
6 tablespoons sunflower seeds
6 teaspoons Bonemeal from a reliable source
(powder or tablets)
6 Vitamin C tablets (.5 grams each)
6 Vitamin E tablets
(200 International Units total)

To these ingredients, add:

6 tablespoons bran flakes

6 teaspoons Kelp powder (or 6-12 Kelp tablets)

Zinc 150 mg

All seeds or tablets should first be crushed in a blender.

Blend ingredients well in a big bowl, stirring until mixture is uniform. To insure freshness and potency, store in a closely covered jar in the refrigerator.

Dosage

It is suggested you take one ounce of this formula daily. Many people sprinkle it on their cottage cheese or yogurt. It may also be taken with soups, hot or cold cereals, vegetable or fruit juices or blended along with a milk shake. For best results, the formula should be a part of a well-balanced diet.

You can buy this amazing formula, pre-mixed, at your local health food store or from reputable mail order supply houses. The formula comes in cans, each about a two-week supply.

Recipes For Using This Healthy Formula

There are many ways to enjoy the benefits of this Dutch doctor's formula. For some suggestions on incorporating this very special supplement into your diet, we have provided recipes. These recipes are only the beginning of what you can do with this formula.

After you read and try these recipes, you will soon be creating new ways for your whole family to benefit from Dr. Rinse's formula.

Healthy Pancakes

1 1/2 cups whole wheat pastry flour

1 teaspoon salt

1 teaspoon brown sugar

2 eggs (optional)

1 cup skim milk

4 tablespoons Dr. Rinse's formula

2 tablespoons safflower oil, for cooking

Combine the flour, salt, brown sugar and the formula. Separately, beat the eggs, add the milk and beat well before mixing with the dry ingredients. If you want a thinner pancake, either omit the eggs or add more milk.

Heat the frying pan, add the oil and proceed to brown the pancakes as you normally would cook them.

Fruity Shake

1 cup fruit of your choice — cantaloupe or strawberries are good choices

1/2 cup plain yogurt

2 teaspoons fructose

1 oz. Dr. Rinse's formula

Combine all ingredients in a blender. Begin mixing on low speed, then gradually blend on high speed until all ingredients are mixed well.

Mocha Cocktails

12 oz. low-fat milk

1 teaspoon instant coffee

1 teaspoon chocolate extract

2 teaspoons honey

1 oz. Dr. Rinse's formula

Combine all ingredients in a blender. Blend at high speed for about one minute before serving.

Q.C.'s Omelette Surprise

2 eggs

1/4 cup low-fat milk

Pinch of chives

2 teaspoons Dr. Rinse's formula

1 teaspoon safflower oil, for cooking.

Pepper, to taste

Filling:

Tomatoes and onions, diced

Mozzarella Cheese

Mushrooms

Beat the eggs. Add the milk, chives and formula. Add pepper to taste. Warm the oil in a frying pan. Pour in the eggs and allow them to partially cook.

When they begin to solidify, gently lift the edges with a spatula, allowing the uncooked portion to fully cook.

Before you fold the omelette, place the filling ingredients on the eggs. Turn off the heat. Cover the pan to allow the cheese to melt. Fold and serve.

Quincy's Peanut Butter Spread

1 tablespoon peanut butter
1 tablespoon brown sugar
1 tablespoon Dr. Rinse's formula
2 tablespoons boiling water

Mix ingredients well. Use this healthy spread as you would regular peanut butter.

Andrew's Apple Butter Spread

6 tablespoons apple butter
1/4 tablespoon cinnamon
1 oz. Dr. Rinse's formula

In a small bowl, combine ingredients and mix thoroughly. You can either use this as a spread or eat it as pudding. Either way, it is delicious and healthy.

Hot Chocolate Deluxe (serves four)

3 cups hot chocolate drink
1 teaspoon vanilla extract
2 oz. Dr. Rinse's formula

Prepare the hot chocolate drink as package indicates. Then pour into a blender and add the remaining ingredients. Blend at high speed for about a minute and a half before serving.

Teri's Bran Muffins

10 tablespoons Dr. Rinse's formula
1 cup whole wheat flour
1 1/2 cups coarse bran
1 egg
1/3 cup blackstrap molasses
1/2 teaspoon grated orange rind
1 teaspoon baking sofa
1/2 teaspoon cinnamon
Pinch of nutmeg
1/2 cup raisins which have been soaked in 3/4 cup water (save the water)

Combine flour, bran, pre-mixed formula, baking soda, cinnamon, orange rind and nutmeg. Beat in the egg and the water in which the raisins were soaking. Add the molasses. Combine well. Blend in the raisins.

Bake in buttered muffin tins for twenty minutes in 330 degree pre-heated oven.

Naturally Fermented Tea Drinks: The Alternative To Harsh Drugs

Utte Sondermann suffered from arthritis in her wrists for several years. She was only in her late 20s;

too young, she thought, to be facing the problem of arthritis.

The pain developed suddenly. "One day my wrists had become swollen and inflamed. It was, without a doubt, the most excruciating pain I have ever known." It soon spread to other joints.

She sought help through a variety of means, including gold shots. Just about everything worked temporarily but the arthritis would always return with a vengeance. "No medical treatment could effectively reduce the pain," she said.

Then a friend recommended a naturally fermented tea drink. He had used it for a health problem and found considerable relief.

"I take three glasses daily," Utte said. "Now I feel wonderful. I can walk up and down the steps again." Then she said with a smile, "And I can dance with my husband once more."

Tea drinks may be effective on arthritis pain through the elimination of toxins from the body. But these drinks, which are gaining popularity all across Europe, do so much more than that. They work on a variety of conditions by releasing the body's naturally-potent healing powers. Because of this, there are no adverse side effects, as there often are with synthetic arthritis drugs.

Take the health problem of Klaus Ballausen. To look at this 33-year-old man today, you would never suspect that he had spent many years seriously ill. This man makes his living as a carpenter, a physically demanding job. It wasn't too long ago that he thought he would never work again.

"I wasn't always this healthy," Klaus explained. His illness developed "out of the blue," he said. He went from doctor to doctor, but not one could discover what was wrong.

A blood test finally indicated he suffered from an inflammation of the abdomen. Klaus said that surgery, at first, brought much relief. "I was just thankful that it was not cancer," he recalled.

But his good health was short-lived. "The doctors had me taking 25 mg. of cortisone daily — an extraordinarily high dosage," Klaus recalled. Because of this treatment, Klaus' face swelled.

Despite the hundreds of tablets the doctors administered, this young man's condition did not improve. In fact, he seemed to be constantly fighting high fevers and headaches. He would also break out in cold sweats.

"My wife was concerned and as exhausted as I was, from caring for me. Unknown to me, she had been researching naturopathic medicine. She suggested that I visit a naturopathic physician. I agreed."

The results of Klaus' visit were truly astonishing.

The doctor recommended that Klaus begin drinking a naturally fermented tea drink. "After just nine glasses, three short days," Klaus said, "my headaches disappeared and my fever subsided.

" And with every single glass, my condition improved. Within several months, all my troubles were gone. Today, I once again work at my trade of carpentry. I even jog now. That tea drink has given me a new lease on life."

Studies indicate that natural tea drinks may have a special beneficial effect on the elderly. Older people who drink these teas daily all reported similar rejuvenating experiences. Their hair, which had been thin and gray for years, began growing back thick and dark. Many people who had skin that sagged and wrinkled, experienced tightening and gained a smoother, more youthful appearance due to the wonderful effects of these drinks. Every older person, moreover, said they felt younger and happier since they had been drinking the beverage.

The Discovery

Dr. Rudolf Sklenar, a German medical doctor, is credited with the modern renaissance of the tea drinks as a natural health treatment. World War II interrupted his medical career but, as it turned out, the war offered him a chance of a lifetime.

While stationed in various parts of Eastern Europe and the Soviet Union as a young medical officer, the doctor began to notice the health of the native peasants, which seemed extremely good. He also observed their custom of drinking a fruity, sparkling drink, unfamiliar to him.

He soon discovered it was a naturally fermented tea drink. The European and Russian peasants began each morning with this beverage, even before they ate their hearty breakfast. They also drank a glass prior to dinner and supper.

These people had very few health problems. It was rare for one of them to come down with a cold. The young doctor thought this was remarkable, because they worked in the fields throughout the year, even in the coldest of weather.

Moreover, these natives lived much longer than people of the more industrialized areas of Europe. It was not at all unusual for them to live active lives well into their 90s and 100s.

As Dr. Sklenar grew to know these people better, he asked more questions about their health and the unusual drink. He soon learned that the two were closely related.

The peasants firmly believed that the tea drink was the reason for their excellent health. Some of the people showed Dr. Sklenar how to grow the plant and to ferment the drink.

At the end of the war, Dr. Sklenar brought the

plant home with him and began making the natural beverage. He systematically administered it to some of his patients, especially those who did not respond to conventional treatment.

The results were amazing. The doctor discovered that the beverage worked well on an array of illnesses and chronic complaints, including migraine headaches, digestive problems, bladder troubles, prostate disorders and many more. Many women who had suffered with monthly problems due to menstrual tension or menopausal difficulties never were bothered with them after using the beverage regularly.

Dr. Sklenar's reputation as a "miracle worker" grew and he gained a world-wide following of patients. When other doctors were unable to alleviate a person's suffering, they referred the patient to Dr. Sklenar, who could help.

The history of naturally fermented tea drinks goes back much farther than Dr. Sklenar's use of it. It dates back to the Orient of ancient times, hundreds of years before the birth of Christ. During the Tsin Dynasty of China—about 221 B.C.—tea drinks were highly popular with royalty, who drank them regularly. These rulers believed that the drinks contained a magical, mystical quality which would give them immortality. The drinks are still widely used today in China for everyday illnesses.

From China, the consumption of these teas progressed to Russia and Eastern Europe. In the 1950s, in fact, naturally fermented tea drinks were the status symbol for the Italian upper classes, who drank the beverages at social functions as well as at home.

Today, these drinks are enjoying unparalleled popularity and are used by the young and old, by the sick and by athletes.

How It Works

While its wondrous effects remained a mystery to primitive civilizations, modern research has studied the drinks and analyzed the components individually. This intensive investigation has proven that they indeed possess highly effective healing powers.

The carbonic acid in the drinks provides the "sparkling taste" which makes them such an enjoyable beverage.

Natural tea drinks contain just the right proportion of components to enable them to attack harmful substances in the body. The beverages break down uric acid and cholesterol into more soluble forms that the body can remove.

For example, gout is caused by a build-up of uric acid. European doctors are now recommending these health beverages both as a preventive and a therapeutic remedy for gout, as well as high blood pressure, arteriosclerosis and age-related complaints.

The glucuronic and lactic acids in the beverages

are the two main active ingredients. They contribute not only to the drinks' cleansing action, but also to its effectiveness in combatting cancer.

Scientific studies say, in fact, that glucuronic acid is the agent responsible for the beverages' cleansing the system of impurities. Once the toxins have been washed from the body, the optimum environment is established for the proper functioning of the body's organs.

When a person drinks these teas, the glucuronic acid in the beverages latches onto the harmful substances in the body and eliminates them from the system. With these "poisonous" substances removed, the body can then concentrate on rebuilding its immune system and processing its stored energy. Thus, it is believed the glucuronic acid plays the most vital role in strengthening the immune system and regulating the body's metabolic processes.

Lactic acid is also essential in rejuvenating the blood and normalizing blood pressure, thus making it a great preventive measure for hypertension.

Moreover, studies have shown that the level of lactic acid is related to the pH level of the blood. A lactic acid deficiency eventually alters the pH level, making the blood more alkaline and more susceptible for the development of cancerous tumors. The pH level is the measure of hydrogen ion concentration present. A pH level of less than 7 is considered acid and above 7 is called alkaline.

Therefore, the beverage's pH level of 3 is of crucial importance in contributing to good health. The pH level of the blood in a young, healthy person tends, on the whole, to be more on the acid side. As a person ages, however, it gradually becomes more alkaline. The average level in the blood of an adult is about 6. If the blood becomes too alkaline, rising to a level of 7.56, it becomes a good setting for the development of tumors and other diseases.

Dr. Veronica Carstens, a medical doctor of great repute and the wife of the former West German president, recommends these tea drinks as a supplement to her cancer patients' regular treatments. "The lactic acid in the naturally fermented drinks is very important to my patient's treatment," she said.

Effectiveness Recognized

The remarkable effectiveness of this new natural therapy has been proven in controlled medical settings. It has brought relief to hundreds of thousands of Europeans who thought their lives would be forever restricted by their illnesses.

The amazing tea drink has won the hearts of those suffering from chronic ailments, such as the many forms of arthritis, as well as the genuine respect of the medical community. Quite an accomplishment for a natural remedy — especially impressive when you consider it has only been on the market for about two years in Europe. But it has been used and tested by

Dr. Sklenar for over 25 years.

Doctors have begun including this therapy as a supplement to their patients' regular treatments. Athletes are using it instead of dangerously strong drugs, to help them perform better. In fact, the German Olympic teams are taking these natural beverages as part of their rigorous training for the prestigious world-wide event. Coaches and trainers of these teams, it is reported, are stunned at the dramatic improvement in their athletic abilities.

The most amazing aspect of the drinks is their naturalness. They agree completely with the body and produce no harmful side effects as so many strong medicines do.

When using strong drugs, their effectiveness wears off after continued use. That is not so with the tea drinks. The powers of this form of natural remedy are never diminished with regular use. In fact, continued usage only produces better results. The longer you drink this natural tea, the better you feel.

Unfortunately, this new natural form of alternative therapy is not available in the United states. You can find these naturally fermented tea beverages only in Europe and other countries.

Herbal Supplements: *The Natural Health Breakthrough*

Ellen K. knocked at the door of Mrs. M's home as

she had done twice monthly for the last couple of years. Mrs. M. answered the door much faster than usual and had a radiant smile on her face. "Come in, come in, Ellen," she exclaimed enthusiastically, "I'll be ready in a minute."

Ellen took 76-year-old Mrs. M. grocery shopping every other week. The elderly lady did not drive and arthritis was slowly taking its toll on her. Even walking around a grocery store was difficult.

About two months previously, Mrs. M. answered the door weaker than usual when Ellen arrived and asked her if she could do the shopping for her. "Every bone in my body aches something terrible," she told her younger friend. Of course, Ellen agreed to do the shopping.

Since that episode, Mrs. M. just had not been herself. She had grown depressed and apathetic about things. In fact, she told Ellen once that she really did not care if she lived or not. "Living involves just so much pain these days," she quietly conceded.

So it took Ellen by surprise when Mrs. M. bustled about her two-bedroom house, searching for her purse. "I'm ready now, dear," the woman said brightly. "I'm sorry to keep you waiting."

Ellen remarked on the changes she noticed in her friend's personality and the apparent improvement in her health. "What have you been doing?" she asked.

The elderly woman went into her kitchen without

answering and came back with three tiny pills. "These have changed my life," Mrs. M. said. "I have just learned about them and I want to tell everyone. Because of this special herbal supplement, my arthritis doesn't bother me as it once did. This is the secret which changed by life."

Food supplements fortified with essential vitamins and carefully blended in an herbal compound have recently been introduced in the United States. One in particular, developed in Denmark by Dr. Fleming Norgaard, M.D., D.D.S., has already helped thousands of Scandinavians overcome many chronic and acute health problems. Many people have found relief from the pain of arthritis and have gained energy and vitality because of this most remarkable supplement.

This new product has helped many who previously had given up all hope of discovering any source of relief for their arthritic condition.

One of these is Pohl Nielson, who as a young man developed what is commonly called "poker spine," and is medically known as Ankylosing Spondylitis. The condition, though painful and inconvenient initially, did not interfere with his daily life.

Pohl's problem progressively worsened, and before too long, he could barely move his back; the vertebrae were fusing together. He spent most of his days in bed, lying flat on his back. He rose only when necessary, usually only to make himself meals.

Among his regrets was the inability to garden. That was his first love. Prior to the worsening of his condition, he had been able to immerse himself in his garden, spending hours among his flowers, enjoying the fragrances, marveling at the splendid colors among the blossoms.

He had heard about the remarkable discovery of herbal supplements and tried one of Dr. Norgaard's tablets. He doubted, at first, that it would be able to help a health problem as serious and involved as his own, but he would try anything that even brought the most remote chance of enabling him to enjoy his flower garden once again.

After several weeks of using the formula, Pohl noticed a slight lessening of his pain. In less than three months, he was able to discontinue his other medications (with the knowledge and consent of his personal physician).

Soon, he was able to stay out of bed for the day and, within a remarkably short period of time, Pohl found himself outside gardening again.

His entire disposition improved because of his increasing good health. Where once he was apathetic, Pohl took a new interest in the outside world. He became an avid reader.

His family doctor could only marvel at the transformation of this once severely handicapped man, saying this gentleman truly had undergone "a miraculous change for the better."

Remarkable Effects In A Short Period of Time

This all-natural herbal supplement appears to work first upon those telltale signs of the aging process — flagging energy, lowered resistance to infections and colds. When people begin to experience these remarkable changes, they acquire an entirely new attitude toward life. Many older people, in fact, express a disbelief at the rapid results they receive. They feel as if they have regained their youth and a second chance at life. The acquire a new-found feeling of vitality in addition to relief from aches, pains and many chronic health conditions.

One woman, amazed at her transformation, wondered out loud "how a 60-year-old body would handle these 17-year-old feelings." Luckily the body, thanks to the herbal supplement, handles the increased feelings of youth. A 70-year-old woman marveled at her physical sense of well-being after taking the supplement for about six weeks. "When I walk down the street now, I'm as light on my feet as if I were 18," she said proudly.

Indeed, natural herbal food supplements appear to work simultaneously on the physical and mental aspects of your health—increasing your physical condition while improving your outlook on life. For many arthritis sufferers, the second effect is equally as important as the first.

True health, after all, does not depend upon only one aspect of life. It is, rather, the reflection of the harmonious workings of all aspects of life. The ability of this new natural therapy to fully benefit the whole individual, and not merely treat a symptom, is the outstanding quality of this formula.

Your Diet: Herbal Supplements Can Help

This unique natural health formula is beneficial for a variety of maladies, especially those related to poor diet, as many physicians say arthritis is.

Most people make an honest attempt to eat properly. However, most of us don't realize the very minute quantities of nutrients which are left in foods after the processing is completed. And processed foods are standard fare these days.

The most common consequence of a deficient diet is fatigue. Who among us has never complained of feeling tired? We've all experienced, at least occasionally, that sensation of dreading even the most minor of tasks, simply because our energy resources seemed depleted.

This is one of the areas in which the herbal supplements work best. Many people receive very positive results within relatively short periods of time. The editor of a prominent Scandinavian health magazine, for example, discovered for himself the revitalizing effects of this natural remedy.

It was early evening and he still had much work to do before the magazine would be ready for the 10 a.m.

deadline the following day. He was already quite tired, having put in ten hours at his job and envisioning at least another six or seven ahead of him.

Being knowledgeable in the healthy ways of reviving sagging energy levels, he shied away from stimulants such as caffeine and other potentially dangerous methods. But the fact remained: he needed a boost.

He knew a friend in the office who was taking the new herbal supplement by Dr. Norgaard and borrowed several tablets. He received an influx of natural energy which enabled him to finish his work more quickly than he expected.

These herbal supplements are not stimulants but a carefully selected blend of several natural herbs which activate your body's internal mechanisms and allow a heightened sense of energy and well being.

Strengthens Immune System

Herbal supplements may also boost your immune system, providing you with extra resistance to colds and infections of just about every kind.

Viruses are especially elusive, according to Dr. Flemming Norgaard, the developer of one of the most popular herbal supplements on the market today. There are so many different forms and there is no effective medication for the viruses.

Many vaccines have not been as successful as

health professionals had originally hoped, because of the microbe's ability to mutate, or to change its composition, which renders the vaccine ineffective.

Viruses, according to Dr. Norgaard, are the most common cause of infection in the upper respiratory area, accounting for about 95 percent of all problems in this region. Therefore, if you could strengthen your immune system, you can increase your protection against the viruses.

Regular use of these new herbal supplements may help you do this. Consider the example of Gerald F., a 62-year-old business executive who could always count on getting at least two serious colds every winter. These colds seemed to linger throughout the entire cold and flu season, invariably costing him several days of work — usually the most critical days. He would miss the signing of an important contract or have to cancel a luncheon appointment with an influential client, due to his colds.

His wife, understanding his plight, bought him a bottle of an herbal supplement. At first, he was hesitant to try it, assuming it would be ineffective. Gerald, however, finally began to use it regularly. His incidence of colds dropped dramatically.

Gerald has been taking the herbal supplement for several years now and has not had a serious cold in that time. When he feels the first symptoms of a cold he immediately takes six tables — twice the normal dosage — for several days. The symptoms usually vanish.

And, because of his improved attendance and dependability in the winter months, Gerald received his long-awaited promotion to vice president.

If you ever feel the symptoms of the cold or flu, double your usual dosage of the herbal supplement immediately. This remarkable natural remedy may be able to stop a cold within ten to twelve hours. Moreover, in these instances, the doctor says, the fatigue which follows the illness, sometimes as troubling as the cold itself, may also be avoided.

Other Viruses Held In Check

Herbal supplements have been known to help reduce the frequency of outbreaks associated with Herpes Simplex I and II. Currently, medical science has not been able to develop a vaccine for this virus. All doctors can hope to do is control the outbreaks of the herpes lesions. For some people, this brings little relief.

For many affected with the Herpes Simplex II virus, no medication seems to help reduce the frequency or severity of the outbreaks. One woman endured almost weekly eruptions of lesions until her physician, having exhausted all other avenues of treatment, recommended an herbal supplement.

As long as she used the natural remedy — without missing any days — she was free of all eruptions. If she skipped taking her three daily pills, however, the herpes returned.

The herbal supplement is not a cure for the virus but rather a way of helping the body resist the virus. Herpes viruses lie dormant within the central nervous system and then emerge during periods of crises or nervousness, which are typically times of lowered immune resistance.

Heart And Circulation May Benefit

The natural ingredients found in the herbal supplement have been reputed, historically, to help strengthen the heart and increase circulation. Many report that dizziness, associated with hardening of the arteries, was relieved with regular use of this amazing product. Several people even said the frequency of their angina pains had been substantially reduced, as well as the severity of the attacks, since they began using the supplement regularly.

These people were most grateful for these outstanding results but were especially thankful they were accomplished without any adverse side effects which, unfortunately, are all too common in the often harsh medication given for these problems.

Menopausal Problems Overcome

Menopause affects women both physically and mentally. It is not surprising then that herbal supplements, with their unique ability to bring mental and physical health into balance, have been able to help women who are going through the change of life.

Many women experience freedom from hot flashes, moodiness and nervousness associated with menopause. And all of this is accomplished without the use of potentially dangerous and often harsh synthetic medications.

These wonderful herbal supplements normalize a woman's system naturally, while increasing her vitality and energy levels.

Not A Placebo Effect

Some may suggest that the wonderful effects experienced by these people are merely the result of the placebo effect. That is, those who expected the herbal supplement to work actually convinced their bodies of this — and their condition improved.

That explanation would not account for the many examples of pets — dogs and cats — benefiting from these wonderful tablets.

A twelve-year-old dog, named Dick, was a member of a French family who ran a small restaurant. He was helped by the herbal supplement.

The dog announced the arrival of new guests with friendly short barks. Those who entered whom he knew were greeted with a loving wag of his tail.

This dog, a long-time family pet, was growing

increasingly decrepit, however. One day, he had to be carried home from a walk. The veterinarian said it was heart degeneration and prescribed some medication but it did not seem to help. The animal's once shiny coat had lost its luster. The pet seemed to lose all interest in his family.

The dog's owner decided to give Dick one table of the herbal supplement every other day. It took only two months before this animal was once again happily greeting the guests at the family's restaurant.

Another family discovered the amazing abilities of the supplement on a stray kitten. They had found this small animal, barely four weeks old. The little kitty seemed quite sickly and could not keep food in her stomach.

The people fed her a crushed herbal blend tablet. Some improvement was noticed after just one tablet. In several days, they gave her another one.

Family members continued this routine daily. very shortly, the kitten improved and was soon eating food on her own. It grew into a beautiful, loving cat.

Another dog was also helped by this natural remedy, although in this case it occurred quite by accident. A 14-year-old Pekinese was near death. Her owner was told the dog might die at any time. Indeed, the animal had refused to eat and had grown extremely apathetic.

One day, the woman dropped an herbal tablet on

the floor. The dog sniffed it and then ate it. After this, the animal's owner continued to give the dog one table daily.

It did not take long for the Pekinese to experience the marvelous effects of the Danish formula. The dog now eats well and has lots of energy, playing fetch and other games with his owner.

Another All Natural Supplement

A newly developed homeopathic composition is being used by top health professionals in Europe with great success. This non-toxic formula includes the ingredients Rhus Toxicodendron D6, Causticum Hahneman D4 and Ferrum Phosphoricum D6.

Perhaps those ingredients do not mean much to you but, as an arthritis sufferer, you may want to look into their use. The tablets produced by this combination are very effective in controlling and eliminating abrupt pain and swelling in the joints — especially joints in the hand, wrist, elbows, ankles and feet.

These tablets have also brought relief for swelling in muscle tissue and connective tissue of the muscle joints, pain associated with back, neck, shoulders and thighs. While it is very effective, this all natural supplement has no side effects.

Available In The U.S.

These remarkable herbal and homeopathic supplements are finally available in the United States. Whether you suffer from arthritis or any other chronic ailment, you owe it to yourself to try these natural remedies. They are fast becoming popular natural supplements with people all across the country. You can purchase these natural food supplements in health food stores as well as select mail order firms.

Epilogue

Good health is not something that just happens to people, as many of us once thought. It takes discipline, hard work and determination. But the rewards are like no other.

That is why more of us are taking direct control of our bodies and learning more about how we can acquire health and how we can maintain it.

This book is intended to help you along the road to good health. It is one resource to use on your journey.

Throughout the volume, we explained how various products may make your quest for robust health easier. You should be able to find all of these products in your local health food store. If your neighborhood outlet does not carry a certain item, ask them to carry it. Most retailers are glad to comply with special requests.

It is not wise to accept substitutes of a similar nature or a product that is "almost as good as" or "cheaper than" something else.

Whatever the product, someone is bound to find a way to imitate it or produce it cheaper. Very often, this is done at the expense of quality.

Synthetic or chemically fertilized products are often substituted for natural or organic products. These manufacturers try to tell us they are just as good as the original, yet it has been proven there are great differences between these items. Why accept second best when it comes to your health?

We hope that *Breakthroughs In Arthritis* benefits your health. Please let us know your experiences with the suggestions we offer.

May good health be yours.

Appendix 1

We have talked about the importance of a proper diet in controlling arthritis. This section of the book provides you with recipes for healthy, tasty foods which arthritics may eat. While you may discover you need to restrict your diet in order to ease your arthritis pain, that does not mean you have to eat boring foods. On the contrary, the ideas for meals which we present here need only be a starting point. Use your creativity — based on your personal tastes — and make your meals delicious and healthy.

BREAKFAST DISHES

Stewed Apples With Honey

4 oz. apples

1 oz. honey

1/2 cup water

Peel and slice the apples. Put the honey and water into a saucepan and stir over low heat until the honey is dissolved.

Add the apples, cover the pan and allow to cook slowly until the fruit becomes tender.

Cool the mixture and spoon into a serving dish. Chill and serve.

Muesli

2 tablespoons quick cooking rolled oats

6 tablespoons water

2 large apples

1 tablespoon plain yogurt

Honey

The following may be added to the recipe according to your tastes:

Raisins	Bananas	Peaches
Apricots	Pears	Grapes

Soak the oats in the water overnight. Wash and grate the apples, then mix with the oats. Add yogurt. Add honey and other ingredients to taste.

Granola Cereal

1/4 cup raisins

8 cups rolled oats

3 large dates

2 large bananas

1 tablespoon vanilla

2 teaspoons cinnamon

1/2 cup raw, unsalted sunflower seeds

1 cup chopped walnuts, hazelnuts, pine nuts and almonds

Soak raisins and dates in a half-cup of water until they are plump. Mash the plump dates and raisins with the bananas. Stir in the vanilla.

Separately, mix the oats, sunflower seeds, nuts

and cinnamon. Add to the banana mixture. Spread out on two cookie sheets and bake at 200 degrees until light brown and dry. Store in a dry place.

SOUPS

Onion Soup

3 Spanish onions
5 cups water
2 small onions
1 oz. butter
1/2 cup skim milk
Sea salt
1 1/2 oz. whole wheat flour

Peel and slice onions. Place onions and butter in a covered saucepan and cook for five minutes. Add water and sea salt.

Boil until onions are very tender. Mix flour with skimmed milk, add to the soup. Boil well. Season to taste.

Cabbage Soup

1 large head of cabbage
4 large carrots, sliced
2 cloves garlic
2 turnips, sliced
1 leek, sliced
5 cups water
Chopped parsley
2 teaspoons sea salt

Shred cabbage. Boil water, add all vegetables and sea salt. Simmer for several hours (not more than three).

A half-hour prior to serving, add parsley and cloves of chopped garlic.

FISH

Fish Casserole

16 oz. white fish, cooked in skim milk

2 tablespoons plain yogurt

2 tablespoons skim milk

1 lb. mashed potatoes

1 egg, beaten

1 oz. butter

Sea salt and pepper

2 tablespoons yogurt

Lightly oil a casserole dish that can go into the broiler. Mix fish with milk and yogurt. Season with pepper and sea salt.

Mix mashed potatoes with egg and milk. Season and place over fish. With a fork, poke holes in casserole.

Cover casserole and place in a preheated oven at 350 degrees. Bake for 20 minutes. Remove from oven, dot with butter and place under the broiler to brown.

Baked Haddock

1 large haddock
2 oz. butter
1 egg
1/4 teaspoon pepper
1 tablespoon finely-chopped parsley
1 tablespoon finely-chopped onion
1 1/2 oz. whole wheat bread crumbs
1/4 teaspoon sea salt

Prepare haddock for stuffing. Place bread crumbs into a bowl along with butter, parsley, onion, sea salt and pepper. Mix well.

Beat egg and mix it into the other ingredients. Press this stuffing into the fish and close the end with a skewer.

Place the fish in a buttered baking pan, dust with a little flour and dot with butter.

Bake in a preheated oven at 350 degrees for 20 to 30 minutes.

Salmon Steaks

4 salmon steaks
1 shallot, chopped
Finely-chopped parsley
Apple cider vinegar
Sea salt
Pepper

Place steaks in a buttered baking dish, season with shallot, parsley, salt, pepper and vinegar. Cover and cook in a preheated oven at 425 degrees for 10 to 15 minutes.

Steamed Trout

4 trout, cleaned

4 tablespoons apple cider vinegar

1 tablespoon chopped parsley

1 teaspoon dried thyme

For the sauce:

1/2 cup plain yogurt

3 tablespoons apple cider vinegar

1/2 teaspoon dried tarragon

1 teaspoon chives

2 teaspoon grated horseradish

Place trout on a large sheet of aluminum foil, sprinkle with vinegar, parsley and thyme. Wrap foil around the fish and place between two plates. Stand them in a pan of boiling water. Steam until fish is tender, about 10 to 15 minutes.

For the sauce:

Place the yogurt, horseradish, tarragon, chives and vinegar into the top of a double boiler and allow to cook for several minutes. The sauce will get hot and creamy. Pour the sauce over the trout and serve immediately.

CHICKEN DISHES

Orange-Rice Chicken

2 boneless chicken breasts, cubed
2 tablespoons vegetable oil
2 tablespoons butter
1/2 cup celery, cut in small pieces
2 cups Mandarin oranges, drained
2 cups cooked rice
1/4 cup sliced almonds

Saute chicken in vegetable oil in a large skillet until tender. Remove from skillet and set aside. In the same skillet, melt butter and saute celery. Then stir in the orange slices, chicken, rice and almonds. Toss together until all ingredients are heated and serve.

Chicken Teri

2 boneless chicken breasts, cut into one-inch strips
1/2 medium sweet red pepper —or —
1/4 medium green pepper, cut into strips
1/2 cup chopped onions
1/2 large crushed garlic clove
1/4 cup plain, low-fat yogurt
Shredded lettuce
1 fresh tomato, chopped
1 oz. butter, for cooking

For marinade:

1 tablespoon apple cider vinegar

1/2 tablespoon chili powder

1/2 teaspoon dried oregano

1/4 teaspoon dry mustard

Dash of cayenne

1/4 cup water

1/3 teaspoon garlic powder

Garnish:

Chopped onions and jalepeno peppers

Place chicken in a large shallow pan. Mix together all marinade ingredients. Pour over chicken and allow to marinate in the refrigerator for at least two hours.

In a large skillet, quickly saute onions and pepper strips. Remove chicken from marinade and place with the sauteed vegetables. Save the marinade.

Cook the chicken until it is firm and white. Pour marinade over chicken and add crushed garlic.

Allow to simmer until the chicken is tender and marinade has just about evaporated.

Arrange lettuce and chopped tomato on a plate. Place meal on top, then spoon yogurt over it. Garnish with onions and jalepeno peppers.

Turkey Sausage

3/4 lb fresh ground turkey

1/2 teaspoon sage

1/2 teaspoon paprika

1/4 teaspoon pepper

1/4 teaspoon fennel seed

1/4 teaspoon thyme

1/8 cup finely chopped parsley

Combine all ingredients into a medium size bowl Mix well. Use in place of sausage on pizza or shape into patties for use as breakfast sausage or in sandwiches. Let your imagination be your guide when trying different ways to serve your healthy "sausage."

MEATLESS DISHES

Vegetable Salad

2 hard-boiled eggs, chopped

2 oz. unpolished rice, cooked

3 small onions, chopped

1 oz. cooked peas

1/2 red pepper, chopped

1/4 cup apple cider vinegar and oil dressing

Mix onions, pepper, peas into rice. Apply dressing. Add eggs last. Serve cold.

Cottage Cheese Fritters

4 oz. whole wheat flour

1 egg, separated

1/2 teaspoon sea salt

5 tablespoons water

8 oz. cottage cheese

Oil, for frying

Sift the flour and salt into a bowl. Make a depression in the center and place the egg yolk into it. Work the flour into the yolk, gradually adding the water. Beat thoroughly.

Beat in the cottage cheese. Whisk the egg white until it just becomes stiff and fold it lightly into the mixture.

Heat oil in a frying pan. Drop in four separate tablespoons of batter and cook over moderate heat until fritters are golden brown. Turn and brown the other side. Remove from oil and drain on paper towel. Repeat with rest of batter.

Makes 16 fritters.

Cabbage Wedge Salad

1/2 lbs. red cabbage, sliced in wedges

1/2 large onion, chopped

1 large unpeeled apple, cored and sliced

2 tablespoons olive oil

1/8 cup apple cider vinegar

2 tablespoons brown sugar

In a 10-inch skillet, saute onion in the olive oil. Then add apple cider vinegar, sugar and apples. Cover with cabbage wedges. Cook slowly, covered, for 10 to 15 minutes. Stir occasionally.

Ginger Broccoli

3 cups fresh broccoli flowerets, cut into bite-size pieces

1/2 teaspoon powdered ginger

2 tablespoons wheat germ

1 clove garlic, minced

1/4 cup butter

1/2 teaspoon salt

Saute garlic in butter until tender. Add wheat germ, ginger and salt. Stir quickly until well mixed and wheat germ is just browned. Be careful not to burn. Add the broccoli and stir well, making sure broccoli pieces are heated and coated.

Nutty Spinach

1/2 tablespoon olive oil

3 tablespoons chopped onion

12 oz. spinach

1 tablespoon pine nuts

1 tablespoon raisins

Vegetable stock to taste

Pinch of salt

Sage, parsley to taste

Saute onions in olive oil. Add spinach and pinch of salt. Simmer uncovered until it becomes slightly soft. Add the pine nuts and raisins. Combine with vegetable stock, if desired. Season with sage and parsley to taste.

Snow Peas A La Rosemary

1/2 tablespoon olive oil
1/2 onion, chopped
7 oz. snow peas
6 tablespoons vegetable stock
Pinch of salt
Parsley and rosemary

Saute onion in olive oil. Add snow peas, stock and salt. Steam in covered pan for a half-hour. Add parsley or rosemary to taste during this time.

Instead of adding salt at the dinner table, use chives, marjoram or thyme.

Marinated Broccoli

1 large head broccoli, flowerets only
1/3 cup herb or balsamic vinegar
1/2 cup safflower oil
1 teaspoon garlic salt
1/2 tablespoon dill weed
1/2 tablespoon honey
1/2 tablespoon soy sauce

Combine all ingredients except broccoli in a bowl. Add broccoli. Marinate for at least 4 hours and not longer than 24. Drain marinade before serving.

Onion Potato Dish

1 lb. potatoes

4 oz. onions

Sea salt and pepper

1 oz. sweet butter

Chopped fresh parsley

Peel potatoes and slice into one-quarter inch thickness. Peel and slice onions. Cover with cold, salted water and bring to a boil.

Simmer five minutes or until cooked. Drain and dry vegetables. Layer potatoes and onions in a lightly buttered frying pan. Season each layer. Dot with butter. Cover pan and cook over medium flame for 10 minutes, shaking pan occasionally to prevent sticking. Serve hot, sprinkled with chopped fresh parsley.

DESSERTS

Baked Apples

Large apples

Sweet butter

Chopped nuts

Honey

Raisins

Core apples, wash them well and fill with nuts and raisins. Place a small piece of butter on top of each and put them in a baking dish. Bake for about one hour in a preheated oven at 350 degrees. Add honey to taste.

Melon Surprise

16 oz. frozen sliced strawberries

8 oz. plain yogurt

Lettuce

3 large cantaloupes

2 cups cream-style cottage cheese

1 cup blueberries

Partially thaw and drain strawberries. Keep one quarter cup of the juice for the syrup of the dressing.

Prepare dressing by mixing yogurt and reserved juice. Cover and chill.

Cut cantaloupes in half, remove the seeds. Using a melon baller, scoop out the pulp.

To make the melon half rest firmly on the salad plate, trim a thin slice from the bottom.

Line the melon shells with lettuce. Place about one-third cup cottage cheese in each melon half. Layer the melon halves with strawberries, then melon balls. Place more cottage cheese, then more strawberries in each melon. Place blueberries in each melon half and top it off with remaining melon balls. Add dressing and serve immediately.

SALAD DRESSINGS

Dill Dressing/Dip

1/2 cup plain yogurt

1/2 tablespoon fresh chives, chopped

1/2 tablespoon dill, chopped

Mix ingredients together. Place in refrigerator and chill for several hours. Serve with vegetables as a dip or double the recipe for a delicious and healthy salad dressing.

Lemon-Herb Dressing

1 teaspoon oil

1 teaspoon lemon juice

1 teaspoon fresh or dried herbs

Onion or garlic to taste

Mix ingredients together. Serve over a salad or fresh vegetables.

Yogurt Dressing

1 tablespoon apple cider vinegar

1 teaspoon caraway seeds

1 teaspoon mustard

1/2 teaspoon salt

1/8 teaspoon garlic salt

1 cup plain yogurt

Combine vinegar and all ingredients except yogurt. Fold in yogurt slowly. Cover and chill for several hours before serving.

Tomato-Lemon Dressing

2 cups tomato juice

1/2 cup lemon juice

Pinch of sugar

Herbs to taste

Mix all ingredients and chill for several hours before serving on your favorite salad.

Nutty Dressing

1 cup chopped pine nuts

1/2 cup olive oil

6 tablespoons tarragon vinegar

1/2 teaspoon grated lemon peel

1/2 teaspoon salt

Dash of nutmeg

Combine all ingredients. Serve over a lettuce salad or over fresh vegetables.

Appendix 2
Glossary of Terms

Analgesic	A pain-killing substance or drug.
Ankylosing Spondylitis	Also called *Mary Strumpell Disease* or "poker spine." It is a condition in which the vertebrae of the back gradually fuse.
Arthritis	A term which includes many different types of ailments affecting the joints and their surrounding areas. The term refers to such common conditions as bursitis, carpal tunnel syndrome and gout.
Auto-Immune Disease	An ailment in which the body's cells attack normal, healthy parts of the body, mistakenly identifying them as foreign invaders.
Bunion	A form of bursitis found on the toes and indicating degenerative changes occurring in the bone.

Bursa	Small pouch in certain joints filled with a gummy fluid, designed to provide extra protection to the body's tissues.
Bursitis	An inflammation of the bursa, the small sac located between the tendon and bone in certain joints.
Capsaicin	The active, natural ingredient found in chili peppers and cayenne which may be beneficial to the arthritis sufferer in helping alleviate the sensation of pain.
Carpel Tunnel Syndrome	Characterized by pain when the wrist is moved and usually affecting the middle three fingers of the hand with a tingling or numbing sensation. A form of tenosynovitis.
Cartilage	An elastic tissue which creates a surface for the joints to slide with the least amount of friction possible.

Cervical Spondylosis	A form of osteoarthritis in which the disc spaces between the vertebrae become compressed. Symptoms include shooting pain from the back of the neck to the head. The pain may even radiate to the hand and accompany a weakness in the arm.
EPA or Eicosapentaenoic Acid	An essential fatty acid, the main source of which is fish. Found to be helpful in easing the symptoms of arthritis, as well as being a natural aid to the heart.
Essential Fatty Acids	Originally called Vitamin F and needed by the human body for proper health. The main sources are vegetable and seed oils.
Flaxseed (Linseed) Oil	A golden vegetable oil, cold-pressed, unrefined rich in linoleic and linolenic acids and may be valuable as a way to reduce the swelling and pain of arthritis.

Gout	A condition related to arthritis and affecting the big toe. Research indicates it is caused by a high level of uric acid in the system. Eating an excess of meats or an overconsumption of alcohol may lead to this condition.
Heberden's Nodes	Small, bony, visible spurs of extra calcium at the end of the finger joints, formed by the body in an attempt to protect the joints.
Hydrotherapy	The treatment of a condition by the application of water, either alternating hot and cold or only using a single type.
Joint Mouse	An osteophyte — or small bony spur — which has broken off and moves about freely inside the joint.
Juvenile Rheumatoid Arthritis	A version of rheumatoid arthritis affecting children which produces many of the same symptoms as adults develop. The cause is unknown.

Nightshade Foods	A family of foods, including potatoes, tomatoes, eggplant, peppers and tobacco which initiates the production of solanine that festers in the joints and muscles. This eventually lowers the body's resistance and may prompt the onset of arthritis.
Osteoarthritis	Most common type of arthritis and usually referred to as the result of "wear and tear" on the joints. Characterized by pain and stiffness in the joints.
Osteophyte	Small bony spur which forms inside the joints by laying down extra calcium at the outer edges of the bones, in an attempt to protect the joint.
Passive Mobilization	One of the first exercises suggested for a joint affected by bursitis. Involves a person gently moving the joint of another who has bursitis.

Poultice	A soft, usually heated, cloth, applied to a sore area or lesion. Many times it is medicated with an herbal preparation.
Pseudogout	Also called chomdrocalcinosis, this condition is related to gout but is the result of calcium salt crystals which have been deposited in the joints. It affects the larger joints, most often the knee.
Psoriatic Arthritis	The person develops psoriasis as well as chronically inflamed joints. Was not recognized as a separate condition until the 1920s.
Reiter's Syndrome	A fairly rare combination of arthritis, conjunctivitis, redness and discharge at the opening of the penis, inflammation of the bladder, a rash on the hands and feet, and painless mouth ulcers.
Rheumatoid Arthritis	A systemic illness affecting not only the joints but also the entire body. Symptoms include fever, chills, loss of appetite and weight, and fatigue.

Still's Disease	A form of juvenile rheumatoid arthritis with major symptoms of high temperature, rash and swelling of the lymph nodes. Joints appear to be unaffected, especially in the early stages of the disease.
Substance P	The neurological transmitter by which capsaicin, an ingredient in chili peppers and cayenne, suppresses pain.
Synovial Membrane	The substance which surrounds and protects the joints and provides lubricating fluid. This allows the ends of the bones to work properly.
Systemic Lupus Erythematosus	A disease, related to arthritis, in which the body attacks its own healthy tissue, which may affect any or all the body. Joint pain is common with this condition.
Tenosynovitis	An inflammation of the tube through which the tendons pass, usually the result of trauma.

Tophi	Uric acid crystals which have collected over several years and form visible nodules just below the surface of the skin. Most often they are found in the elbows and hands.
Uric Acid	A substance associated with the onset of gout, which is found in a number of foods, especially meat and alcohol. The body, though, does produce a certain amount of uric acid itself.

Appendix 3

Clay Resources

The Three Sheaves Company
16 Hudson Street
New York, New York 10013

Weleda
841 S. Main Street
Spring Valley, New York 10977

Appendix 4

Arthritis Foundation Chapters

Alabama

Alabama Chapter
13 Office Park Circle, Room 14
Birmingham, Alabama 35223
(205) 870-4700

South Alabama Chapter
304 Little Flower Avenue
Mobile, Alabama 36606
(205) 471-1725

Arizona

Central Arizona Chapter
2102 W. Indian School Road Suite 9
Phoenix, Arizona 85015
(602) 264-7679

Southern Arizona Chapter
4520 E. Grant Road
Tucson, Arizona 85712
(602) 326-2811

Arkansas

Arkansas Chapter
6213 Lee Avenue
Little Rock, Arkansas 72205
(501) 664-7242

California

Northeastern California Division
1722 "J" Street Suite 321
Sacramento, California 95814
(916) 446-7246

Northern California Chapter
203 Willow Street Suite 201
San Francisco, California 94109

San Diego Area Chapter
6145 Mission Gorge Road Suite 10
San Diego, California 92120
(619) 280-0304

Southern California Chapter
4311 Wilshire Boulevard
Los Angeles, California 90010
(213) 938-6111

Colorado

Rocky Mountain Chapter
234 Columbine Street Suite 210
P.O. Box 6919
Denver, Colorado 80206
(303) 399-5065

Connecticut

Connecticut Chapter
370 Silas Deane Highway
Weathersfield, Connecticut 06109
(203) 563-1177

Delaware

Delaware Chapter
234 Philadelphia Pike Suite 1
Wilmington, Delaware 19809
(302) 764-8254

District of Columbia

Metropolitan Washington Chapter
1901 Ft. Myer Drive Suite 507
Arlington, Virginia 22209
(703) 276-7555

Florida

Florida Chapter
3205 Manatee Avenue, West
Bradenton, Florida 33505
(813) 748-1300

Georgia

Georgia Chapter
1340 Spring Street NW
Atlanta, Georgia 30309
(404) 873-3240
1-800-282-7023

Hawaii

Hawaii Chapter
200 North Vineyard Suite 503
Honolulu, Hawaii 96817
(808) 523-7561

Idaho

Idaho Chapter
700 Robbins Road Suite 1
Boise, Idaho 83702
(208) 344-7102

Illinois

Central Illinois Chapter
Allied Agencies Center
320 East Armstrong Avenue Room 102
Peoria, Illinois 61603
(309) 672-6337

Illinois Chapter
79 West Monroe Suite 1120
Chicago, Illinois 60603
(312) 782-1367

Indiana

Indiana Chapter
1010 East 86th Street
Indianapolis, Indiana 46240
(317) 844-3341

Iowa

Iowa Chapter
1501 Ingersoll Avenue
Suite 101
Des Moines, Iowa 50309
(515) 243-6259

Kansas

Kansas Chapter
1602 East Waterman
Wichita, Kansas 67211
(316) 263-0116

Kentucky

Kentucky Chapter
1381 Bardstown Road
Louisville, Kentucky 40204
(502) 459-6460

Louisiana

Louisiana Chapter
4700 Dryades
New Orleans, Louisiana 70115
(504) 897-1338

Maine

Maine Chapter
37 Mill Street
Brunswick, Maine 04011
(207) 729-4453

Maryland

Maryland Chapter
12 West 25th Street
Baltimore, Maryland 21218
(301) 366-0923

Massachusetts

Massachusetts Chapter
59 Temple Place
Boston, Massachusetts 02111
(617) 542-6535

Michigan

Michigan Chapter
23400 Michigan Avenue Suite 605
Dearborn, Michigan 48124
(313) 561-9096

Minnesota

Minnesota Chapter
122 West Franklin Suite 440
Minneapolis, Minnesota 55404
(612) 874-1201

Mississippi

Mississippi Chapter
6055 Ridgewood Road
Jackson, Mississippi 39211
(601) 956-3371

Missouri

Eastern Missouri Chapter
7315 Manchester
St. Louis, Missouri 63143
(314) 644-3488

Western Missouri Greater Kansas City Chapter
8301 State Line Suite 117
Kansas City, Missouri 64114
(816) 361-7002

Montana

Montana Chapter
P.O. Box 20994
Billings, Montana 59102
(406) 248-7602

Nebraska

Nebraska Chapter
2229 North 91st Court #33
Omaha, Nebraska 68134
(402) 391-8000

Nevada

Nevada Chapter
3160 South Valley View Blvd. Suite 107A
Las Vegas, Nevada 89102
(702) 367-1626

New Hampshire
New Hampshire Chapter
P.O. Box 369
35 Pleasant Street
Concord, New Hampshire 03301
(603 224-9322

New Jersey

New Jersey Chapter
15 Prospect Lane
Colonia, New Jersey 07067
(201) 388-0744

New Mexico

New Mexico Chapter
5112 Grand Avenue NE
Albuquerque, New Mexico 87108

New York

Genesee Valley Chapter
973 East Avenue
Rochester, New York 14607
(716) 271-3540

Long Island Division
501 Walt Whitman Road
Melville, New York 11747
(516) 459-5082

Northeastern New York Chapter
1237 Central Avenue
Albany, New York 12205
(518) 459-5082

Western New York Chapter
1370 Niagara Falls Blvd.
Tonawanda, New York 14150
(716) 837-8600

North Carolina

North Carolina Chapter
P.O. Box 2505
3115 Guess Road
Durham, North Carolina 27705
(919) 477-0286

North Dakota

Dakota Chapter
1402 North 39th Street
Fargo, North Dakota 58102
(701) 282-3653

Ohio

Central Ohio Chapter
2501 North Star Road
Columbus, Ohio 43221
(614) 488-0777

Northeastern Ohio Chapter
11416 Bellflower Road
Cleveland, Ohio 44106
(216) 791-1310

Northwestern Ohio Chapter
4447 Talmadge Road
Toledo, Ohio 43623
(419) 473-3349

Southwestern Ohio Chapter
2400 Reading Road
Cincinnati, Ohio 45202
(513) 721-1027

Oklahoma

Eastern Oklahoma Chapter
2816 East 51st Street
Suite 120
Tulsa, Oklahoma 74105
(918) 743-4526

Oregon

Oregon Chapter
Barbur Blvd. Plaza
4445 SW Barbur Blvd.
Portland, Oregon 97201
(503) 222-7246

Pennsylvania

Central Pennsylvania Chapter
P.O. Box 668
2019 Chestnut Street
Camp Hill, Pennsylvania 17011
(717) 763-0900

Eastern Pennsylvania Chapter
311 South Juniper Street
Suite 201
Philadelphia, Pennsylvania 19107
(215) 735-5272

Western Pennsylvania Chapter
428 Forbes Avenue Suite 2401
Pittsburgh, Pennsylvania 15219
(412) 566-1645

Rhode Island

Rhode Island Chapter
850 Waterman Avenue
E. Providence, Rhode Island 02914
(401) 434-5792

South Carolina

South Carolina Chapter
1802 Sumter Street
Columbia, South Carolina 29201
(803) 254-6702

South Dakota
See North Dakota

Tennessee

Middle-Eastern Tennessee Division
210 25th Avenue North, #1202
Nashville, Tennessee 37203
(615) 329-3431

West Tennessee Chapter
2600 Poplar Avenue Suite 200
Memphis, Tennessee 38112
(901) 452-4482

Texas

North Texas Chapter
6300 Harry Hines Blvd. Suite 211
Exchange Park, Treadway Plaza
Dallas, Texas 75235
(214) 956-7771

Northwest Texas Chapter
3145 McCart Avenue
Fort Worth, Texas 78204
(817) 926-7733

South Central Texas Chapter
503 South Main Street
San Antonio, Texas 78204
(512) 224-4857

Texas Gulf Coast Chapter
9111-A Katy Freeway Suite 210
Houston, Texas 77024
(713) 468-6572

West Texas Chapter
2317 34th Street
Lubbock, Texas 79411
(806) 793-3273

Utah

Utah Chapter
Graystone Plaza #15
1174 E. 2700 South
Salt Lake City, Utah 84106
(801) 486-4993

Vermont

Vermont Chapter
Richardson Place Suite 3F
2 Church Street
Burlington, Vermont 05401
(802) 864-4988

Virginia

Virginia Chapter
1900 Byrd Avenue Suite 100
P.O. Box 6772
Richmond, Virginia 23230
(804) 282-5491

Washington

Western Washington Chapter
726 Broadway Suite 103
Seattle, Washington 98122
(206) 324-9940

West Virginia

West Virginia Chapter
P.O. Box 8473
440 Fourth Avenue
South Charleston, West Virginia 25303
(304) 744-3042

Wisconsin

Wisconsin Chapter
1442 North Farwell Avenue Suite 508
Milwaukee, Wisconsin 53202
(414) 276-0490

Wyoming
See Colorado

Appendix 5
Bibliography of Selected References

Airola, N.D., Ph. D., Paavo, *How To Get Well,* Health Plus Publishers, Phoenix, Arizona, 1974.

Alexander, Dale, *Arthritis and Commonsense,* Simon And Schuster, New York, 1981.

Cooper, Jean, *The Food Pharmacy,* Bantam Books, New York, 1988.

Fischer, William L., *How To Fight Cancer and Win,* Fischer Publishing Co., Canfield, Ohio, 1987.

Fischer, William L., *Miracle Healing Through Nature's Pharmacy,* Fischer Publishing Co., Canfield, Ohio, 1986.

Fredericks, Ph.D., Carlton, *Arthritis: Don't Learn to Live With It,* Grosset and Dunlap, New York, 1981.

Heinerman, John, Heinerman's *Encyclopedia of Fruits, Vegetables and Herbs,* Parker Publishing Co., New York, 1988.

Jarvis, M.D., D.C., *Arthritis and Folk Medicine,* Pan Books, London, 1972.

Jensen, Bernard, Ph.D., *Arthritis, Rheumatism and Osteoporosis,* Dr. Bernard Jensen, Publisher, Escondido, California, 1986.

Jensen, Bernard, Ph.D., *Nature Has A Remedy,* Dr. Bernard Jensen, Publisher, Escondido, California, 1984.

Keough, Carol, *Natural Relief For Arthritis,* Rodale Press, Emmaus, Pennsylvania, 1983.

Lee, R.Ph., Ph.D., *The Book of Raw Fruit and Vegetable Juices and Drinks,* Keats Publishing, Inc., New Canaan, Connecticut, 1982.

Long, Ph.D., Ruth Yale, *A Basic Diet Plan and Use of Food Supplements,* Nutrition Education Association, Inc., Houston, Texas, 1983.

Arthritis and Nutrition, Nutritional Education Association, Inc., Houston, Texas, 1983.

McDougall, John A., M.D., *McDougall's Medicine: A Challenging Second Opinion,* New Century Publishers, Inc., Piscataway, New Jersey, 1985.

Mervyn, Leonard, Ph.D., *Thorsons' Complete Guide To Vitamins and Minerals,* Thorsons Publishers, Inc., Rochester, Vermont, 1987.

Rooney, Theodore W., M.D., and Patty Ryan Rooney, *The Arthritis Handbook,* Ballentine Books, New York, 1985.

Scala, James, M.D., *The Arthritis Relief Diet,* Penguin Books, New York, 1987.

Trattler, Ross, M.D., *Better Health Through Natural Healing,* McGraw-Hill Book Co., New York, 1988.

Walker, N.W., *Raw Vegetable Juices,* The Berkeley Publishing Group, New York, 1984.

Index

A

alkaline, 41, 139, 175, 176
amino acids, 42, 59, 60, 68
Ankylosing Spondylitis, 21-24, 179
aspirin, 49, 52, 53, 62, 68, 79, 139, 163
atherosclerosis, 96

B

barley, 40-42
beer, 145
bone meal, 162
bone powder, 50, 57, 58, 63
brewer's yeast, 36, 161, 163
bunion's, 156, 157
bursa(e), 4, 9, 146-149
bursitis, 4, 83, 135, 146-150, 153-156, 158

C

cabbage, 124, 140, 150, 154
calcium, 3, 5, 44, 50, 56, 58, 63, 75, 96, 121, 145, 162
capsaicin / capsicum, 38, 39
Carpel Tunnel Syndrome, 24-25
carrot, 42, 44, 45, 46, 79-81, 94, 140
cartilage, 3, 4, 8, 23, 67
celery, 43, 44, 47, 140
chamomile, 85
cherries, 34, 55, 140, 144

Index

chili peppers, 37-39
chlorophyll, 31, 32, 41
Chrohn's Disease, 24
circulation, 90, 104, 125, 127, 129, 130, 131, 160, 185
clay, 46, 123, 124
club moss, 81, 82, 143
cod liver oil, 74-76
colitis, 24
coltsfoot, 154
comfrey, 91, 142, 143, 154
constipation, 131-134, 143
crepitant, 6

D

dandelion, 85, 86, 94
Devil's Claw, 92-94
diabetics, 39, 132
Dr. Rinse Formula, 161, 163, 165-168

E

Eicosapentaenoic Acid (EPA), 29
exercise, 6, 18, 25, 95-97, 102, 104-113, 129, 132, 150-152

F

fatigue, 8, 32, 182, 184
fatty acids, 29-31, 65-71
fermented tea, 168-170, 172, 173, 177
feverfew, 86-88, 94
fiber, 32

Index

flaxseed oil, 31
fruit, 28, 29, 31-36, 42, 44, 53-55, 63, 73-74, 76, 120, 121, 140, 141, 144, 150, 164, 165, 172

G

garlic, 33, 142
gout, 32, 80,82, 91, 135-139, 141-147, 157, 174
grapes, 32, 55, 74, 119-122

H

Herpes Simplex, 185
homeopathic, 117, 188, 189
honey, 32, 50, 58, 61, 62, 74, 81, 83, 133, 166
horsetail, 46, 82, 83, 91, 94
hydrotherapy, 126, 153, 158
hypoglycemics, 39

I

ice, 125, 126, 128, 156
inflammation, 8-11, 21, 24, 30, 42, 61, 82, 86, 92 119, 136, 146-148, 156, 157, 170
immune system, 10, 11, 72, 116, 175, 183

J

juice(s), 33, 34, 39-45, 55, 62, 71, 75, 76, 79-81, 140, 142, 145, 154, 164
joint mouse, 5

Index

K

kidney (s), 67, 82, 119, 138, 143

L

lecithin, 36, 161, 163
linoleic / linolenic acids, 66, 69, 70, 72, 73, 163

M

magnesium, 44, 50
marjoram, 89, 94
menopause, 186

N

Naturalax, 132, 133
nightshade (s), 48, 49, 64

O

obese / obesity, 7, 8
okra, 43, 47
osteoarthritis, 1-9, 12, 68, 80, 82
osteophyte, 5

P

pantothenic acid, 50, 56, 59-62, 161
phosphorus, 44, 45, 50, 121
plaque, 69, 160
polycythemia, 138
potato, 28, 29, 45, 47-49, 64, 150

poultices, 91, 124, 154
propolis, 50, 60, 61, 63
prostaglandin, 30, 67, 72
pseudogout, 145, 146
psoriatic arthritis, 20, 21
purine, 140-142, 145

R

rebounding, 108-116
Reiter's Syndrome, 21
relaxation, 17
Reynaud's Syndrome, 17
Rheumapac, 117-119
rheumatoid arthritis, 2, 8-14, 16, 18, 20, 35, 52, 53, 55-57, 63, 80, 81, 92, 118
rheumatoid arthritis, juvenile, 19
Royal Jelly, 50, 58-60, 63

S

St. John's Wort, 88, 90, 124
solanine, 48
speedwell, 155
Still's Disease, 19
stinging nettle, 84, 90
stress, 10, 13, 14, 16, 18, 111
sunflower oil, 163
synovial membrane, 4, 5, 8, 10, 23
systemic, 8
Systemic Lupus Erythematosis, 20

T

tea, 28, 46,81-85, 90, 91, 143, 144, 154, 168-177
tendon, 4, 5, 9, 24, 25, 146
tophi, 137, 138
toxicity, 49, 55, 48, 75
turmeric, 42, 43

U

uric acid, 32, 136, 138-141, 145, 157, 174

V

vegetable(s), 28, 29, 31-35, 44, 45, 48, 54, 63, 140, 141, 154, 157, 164
veal broth, 47, 48
vinegar, apple cider, 50, 61, 157
vitamin B, 56, 60
vitamin C, 42, 50-55, 62, 148-150, 158, 162, 163
vitamin D, 75, 96
vitamin E, 50, 51, 62, 162, 163
vitamin P, 53-55

W

wheat germ, 132, 162, 163

Y

yarrow, 83, 84

Z

zinc, 50, 57, 60, 63, 162, 164

Other Outstanding Books on Health And Natural Healing From Fischer Publishing

Mysterious Cause Of Illness and How To Overcome Every Disease From Constipation to Cancer
by Jonn Matsen, N.D.

Famed Canadian doctor uncovers the mysterious *REAL* cause of illness—and shows you how to overcome every disease from constipation to cancer. Dr. Matsen's acclaimed food-based "miracle cures" use *no* drugs, *no* surgery. They simply turn on the natural "internal healing power" built into every human body. Here is a safe, easy approach to health and longevity that has cured many "hopeless" cases after conventional medicine has failed! If you read nothing else, read Dr. Matsen's new revelations of secret remedies.

ISBN 0-915421-09-7 ....$16.95

Miraculous Breakthroughs for Prostate and Impotency Problems
by William L. Fischer

Good news for every man who has prostate or occasional impotency problems. This new book describes in detail many of the latest therapeutic discoveries from Europe and America that can prevent, relieve or cure prostate disease, without the agony of prostate surgery. The book also discusses other male problems like testicle diseases, cancer, and the subject of impotency with honesty and sensitivity.

ISBN 0-915421-12-7 ....$18.95

Eye Secrets To Better Sight
by William L. Fischer

This important new book discusses the latest natural treatments for most common eye diseases. The author presents symptoms of various eye conditions from cataracts and glaucoma to macular degeneration, from the rare to the common place. He describes the warning signs of numerous eye problems and how to cope with them successfully. Also covered is the very latest in medical technology and explains how new procedures can cure most common sight defects forever. A must to read for everyone who cares about their eyesight—your window to the world—and that of your loved ones.

ISBN 0-915421-14-3 ....$16.95

Secrets To A Healthy Heart And Low Cholesterol
by William L. Fischer

This book can be your valued partner in lowering or maintaining your cholesterol level. Learn about cholesterol, what it does, how it works and why too much is dangerous. It shows you how to take positive steps in improving your current situation and maintaining it for life long health. Hardening of the arteries, or atherosclerosis, is also discussed in detail. It gives no warning signals until it is almost too late. There are effective measures you can take to help delay, prevent and reverse this very serious health problem. Included is also the world famous scientific breakthrough formula by Prof. Norgaard, M.D., D.D.S. from Denmark that has helped thousands of people overcome their illnesses.

ISBN 0-915421-13-5 ....$16.95

The Romance Of Creative Healthy Cookery
by William and Trudy Fischer

We know you'll fall in love with this book because over 800,000 European women with osteoporosis-type conditions have already greatly benefited. All of the recipes are time-tested and medically endorsed. These new inventive dishes were created by health minded experts and nutritionally oriented chefs and have been adapted for ingredients that can be easily purchased at your local grocery store. The book includes calcium-rich recipes to fight or prevent osteoporosis, nutritious meals for the whole family, budget dishes fit for royalty and think light...cook light...eat light recipes everybody will enjoy.

ISBN 0-915421-11-9 ....$18.95

Breakthrough In Arthritis
by William Fischer

If you thought there was nothing you could do for your painful condition, you need to read this book and discover freedom from arthritic pain. Learn more about the complex of nearly one hundred often crippling diseases called arthritis, such as rheumatism, bursitis, gout, carpel tunnel syndrome and more. Sound, natural, safe remedies are offered in detail. Also described in this book is the newest breakthrough formula of a leading world authority on arthritic pain.

ISBN 0-915421-15-1 ....$16.95

How To Fight Cancer And Win by William L. Fischer

It clearly spells out real cancer preventives and cures, many never before published, with strong scientific documentation and stories of miraculous cures. They are all presented in a concise, easy-to-understand style. You can put this vast knowledge into practice to ensure that this deadly disease never strikes home.

ISBN 0-915421-07-0 . . . .$16.95

Shipping/Handling $4.00 for one book.
Additional books $1.00 each.

Fischer Publishing
Box 368
Canfield, Ohio 44406
(216) 533-1232